500 BEAUTY SOLUTIONS

*E*xpert advice on
hair and nail care—
what to buy and how
to use it!

EDITED BY BETH BARRICK-HICKEY

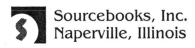

Sourcebooks, Inc.
Naperville, Illinois

Published by: **Sourcebooks** Trade
A Division of Sourcebooks, Inc.
P.O. Box 372, Naperville, Illinois, 60566
(708) 961-2161
FAX: 708-961-2168

This publication is designed to provide accurate and authoritative information in regard to the subject matter covered. It is sold with the understanding that the publisher is not engaged in rendering legal, accounting, or other professional service. If legal advice or other expert assistance is required, the services of a competent professional person should be sought.

From a Declaration of Principles Jointly Adopted by a Committee of the American Bar Association and a Committee of Publishers and Assn.

Library of Congress Cataloging-in-Publication Data
Barrick-Hickey, Beth
    500 beauty solutions / Beth Barrick-Hickey.
        p. cm.
    Includes index.
    ISBN 0-942061-78-0 : $8.95
    1. Beauty. Personal.   I. Title.
RA778.B234   1993
646.7'042--dc20   93-30179
                                                        CIP

Printed and bound in the United States of America.
10 9 8 7 6 5 4 3 2 1

Contents

Chapter **1** – Shampoo To Maintain Your Mane...... **8**

Chapter **2** – Treat Those Tresses **22**

Chapter **3** – Spritz, Sprays, Shiners 'N Gels **38**

Chapter **4** – Tools Of The Trade **56**

Chapter **5** – Plug It In **74**

Chapter **6** – Curl Talk **94**

Chapter **7** – For Women Of Color **114**

Chapter **8** – Hair Color Cues **138**

Chapter **9** – Nail It **158**

Chapter **10** – Skin Care and Hair Removal.......... **192**

References **202**

Glossary **203**

Index **219**

Acknowledgments

This book represents a collaborative effort on the part of many people, from salon owners and salon professionals to the merchandising staff at Sally Beauty Supply.

Credit belongs to Susan Walker, vice president of merchandising for Sally Beauty Supply, who gathered together her store managers, merchandisers, support staff and vendors to collect hundreds of professional answers to these beauty questions.

We consulted Dayton Mast, owner of L'Image Salons in Dallas and Jamie Harry, nail technician. Their tips and advice were excellent.

Elaine Dodson, owner of Elaine Dodson's Natural Way of Beauty Salon in Dallas and a pioneer in natural products for the hair, was an invaluable source of information on botanical products and conditioners.

For many of the answers on color, we thank Bob Goehrke, vice president of marketing, and Deanna Bulkley, director of education, both of Clairol Professional; and Joyce Head of L'Oreal. Teri Faulkner, vice president of marketing for Zotos and James W. Viera, creative technical director for L'Oreal, were also most helpful in providing information on shampoos, conditioners, color and perms. For historical information, we thank Myra Hoshowski, principal scientist for Helene Curtis, Inc. Special thanks to Belson Products marketing department for their information on appliances and to Clyde Hammond, Sr., President of Summit Co., for his contributions on Chapter 7, "For Women of Color."

Additional thanks to Carmen Hathaway and Debbie Jones of OrigiNails for assistance on the "Nail It" chapter and to Dallas researchers, Tomarie Miller and Jeanie Collier, for their assistance in developing questions and investigating product information and advice, and to Dr. Jim Albright, professor/advertising and journalism at the University of North Texas, Denton for editing assistance.

A final thank you to the creative sources who were instrumental in helping design a book we hope women around the country will want to own, award-winning graphic designer Bill Ford of Ford and Company in Dallas, illustrator Mark Foltz, and nationally known fashion photographer Charlie Freeman in Dallas, and our beauty and marketing specialists in Dallas and New York, Rosanne Hart and Jane Gyulavary, who conceived the book.

It is our hope that "500 Beauty Solutions" provides quick answers to those perplexing questions you have between salon visits. It's like having your own beauty expert on call 24 hours a day!

– Beth Barrick-Hickey

> *Thank you to my husband, Emmett,*
> *and to my family*
> *for their support, patience and enthusiasm*
> *on the book.*
> —Beth

Introduction

Long before the days of Cleopatra, women regarded hair as their crowning glory. Beauty regimens are as old as time. And if one thing holds true throughout the ages, it is that women will continually seek ways to improve the way they look. As we edge closer to the 21st Century, more and more products fill the shelves of drug stores, grocery stores, salons and beauty supply outlets. The endless array is mind-boggling, overwhelming and confusing at best! What shampoo should you use? What brush won't split ends? Which nail file works best on acrylic nails?

Colorful labels, beautifully illustrated packaging, bold claims, sweepstakes and two-for-one promotions beckon you at every turn as you shop for just the right beauty solution.

"500 Beauty Solutions" is designed to help you cut through the clutter to solve your hair, nail, skin and depilatory concerns. This book answers the questions you may have wanted to ask your stylist. And it will come to the rescue when a beauty crisis erupts at the most inopportune time.

Straight talk is all there is. No weighty technical jargon that requires a chemistry degree. No heavy blocks of copy you must wade through to find a solution.

HOW TO USE THIS BOOK

"500 Beauty Solutions" is the first comprehensive book written for consumers from a professional point of view that gives hair and nail care advice in a quick, easy-to-read format.

You'll discover not only how to solve a problem, but also what specifically to use to solve your problem. Who better than the professionals to give you advice on how to care for your hair, nails and skin?

Most of the products mentioned in this book are available through beauty salons, beauty supply stores or the more than 1,200 Sally Beauty Supply stores throughout the world. Many of the products mentioned are comparable to branded lines available only in salons. What makes the products mentioned in this book unique, in many cases, is that they offer not only professional quality, but also a value. And in these times of growing budgetary concerns, affordability is an important issue.

"500 Beauty Solutions" is divided into 10 chapters, each almost equally devoted to advice and product-specific solutions. Many of the solutions are applicable to all women; however, a special chapter covers the unique needs of women of color. Although the emphasis is on the care of hair and nails, a short chapter has been included on skin care, specifically depilatory products for face and body.

Sprinkled throughout the chapters is FY ⬤ , information that is basic to understanding how to care properly for hair and nails.

As more and more consumers, as well as beauty media, looked to Sally Beauty and other beauty professionals for the answers to their beauty questions, the need for a book that addressed common beauty problems from a professional point of view became obvious.

"Just give me the facts," women would tell us. "I just want to know what to buy that will make my hair look better," they said.

And for the hundreds of women who walk into a Sally Beauty Supply, a drug store, beauty salon or beauty supply to purchase hair and nail care products, the question undoubtedly arises, "There's so much here, where do I begin?"

Start here with "500 Beauty Solutions," the complete guide to all your hair and nail care needs. Pop it into the top drawer of your vanity or wherever you do your hair and nails. Take it with you on vacation, when you travel for business or pleasure. Whatever you do, you won't want to leave home without it!

Shampoo to Maintain your Mane

T he word "shampoo" was born in England when British hairdressers coined the word "shampoo" from the Hindu word "champo" which means "to massage" or "to knead." But, it was not until the 1890s in Germany that the first actual detergent-based shampoo was introduced to the world. Previously, cleansing solutions for the hair were concocted as early as ancient Egyptian times when the Egyptians mixed water and citrus juice to remove the hair's sebum oil.

The modern shampoo business owes its beginning in America to John Breck, who developed various hair and scalp cleansing solutions in hopes of curing his early-onset baldness. Breck first came up with shampoos for normal hair which were popular in beauty salons in the '30s. Later, he developed a complete shampoo line for oily and dry hair. Although he had built an empire of hair care products, Breck was not able to stop his own baldness.

Today, there are hundreds of shampoos available, from expensive brand names lining cosmetic counters of the finest department stores to promotionally priced gallons of shampoo from your local discounter.

Shampoos do more than just clean hair and stimulate the scalp. In your salon, your stylist uses sham-

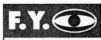

The pH Factor

The term "pH" refers to the balance between acid and alkaline, which must be measured with the presence of water, because dry substances do not have a pH. pH ranges from 0 to 14.0, with 7.0 being neutral, like water. Anything under 7.0 is acid, anything above is alkaline. Human hair seems to like a mildly acid pH level. Although hair has no pH, the scalp and the natural oils which coat the cuticle of the hair do have a pH between 4.5 and 5.5. Shampoos that claim to be pH-balanced usually range from 4.5 to 6.5. Basically, pH-balanced means that the shampoo is gentle, not harsh.

poo to prepare hair for chemical services, such as perms or hair color. Shampoos are also helpful in adding body, texture and shine to hair. Some revive color, while others can strip away styling product build-up or even chlorine from the pool.

The key to selecting the right shampoo for you is the type of hair you have. Is it normal, oily, dry, fine, coarse, or chemically treated? The condition of your hair is important, as well. When visiting your stylist, ask to have your hair analyzed. Your stylist can help you make the right choice.

Q. **Are professional hair care products really different than those found in grocery, drug or department stores?**

A. Yes! There are significant differences in professional products. Some contain higher concentrations of certain ingredients such as protein. A key benefit is that salon or professional products are often developed based on the hairstylist's actual experiences, rather than the manufacturers marketing surveys! Professional shampoos have a pH of 4.5 to 6.5, and emollients and cleansers are blended to break dirt and oil into tiny particles that slide harmlessly off hair and scalp.

2 Q. Is there a shampoo that will make my hair grow faster?

A. No shampoo will grow hair, but there are several that help add fullness and that clean well to keep scalp healthy and which aid in allowing hair to grow faster. John Breck spent much of his career trying to answer that same question. Try Folicure Shampoo or Jheri Redding Professional Prescription Biotin Shampoo.

3 Q. What is an "everyday" shampoo?

A. Although most shampoos are designed to be used everyday, there are some products designated as everyday or lighter formula shampoos. These shampoos are usually milder and have a slightly acid pH level that hair likes. Light formulas are good for fine, wavy or curly hair that is flattened overnight and needs to be fluffed up by shampooing. The most important thing to remember is to choose a shampoo that fits your hair type (normal, oily, dry, permed, colored). Ion Balanced Cleansing Shampoo, Quantum Shampoo, Design Freedom Daily Cleansing Shampoo or Professional Prescription Absolute Shampoo are considered everyday shampoos.

F.Y.⊙

What is Hair?

Hair is made of a strong protein called "Keratin" which contains 21 different amino acids. The hair shaft consists of the cuticle, the cortex and the medulla. The cuticle is the outer layer of the hair shaft, made of multiple layers of translucent cells which overlap each other like shingles on a roof. When the layers are smooth and flat against each other, the hair reflects more light and looks shiny. The middle layer of an individual hair is called the cortex which comprises three quarters of the hairshaft. The pigment, or melanin, gives hair its color and is located in the cortex. There are two types of melanin: eumelanin, black pigment, and pheomelanin, red/yellow pigment. The core of the hair shaft is called the medulla.

4 Q. I have so many different brands of shampoos in my bathroom. Should I use the same brand on my hair everyday or should I alternate them?

A. It's fine to use the same shampoo day after day, as long as you are using the correct shampoo for your hair type. Try using a clarifying shampoo periodically to eliminate any build-up of conditioning and styling products.

5 Q. I love using styling products like mousse and gel to give my hair body, but I don't think my shampoo is getting rid of all that build-up. What should I do?

A. Use a gentle cleansing shampoo routinely once or twice a week. Depending on the build-up, use a deep cleanser or clarifying shampoo. A clarifying shampoo, which contains more detergent than an everyday shampoo, is designed to lightly strip the hair. It usually has a higher pH level, too. Use only as needed and follow with a conditioner. Try Quantum Clarifying, Ion Clarifying Shampoo, Salon Care Ultra Moisturizing Anti Chlorine Shampoo, or Queen Helene RX-18. Use once a week, but never more than twice a week.

6 Q. What ingredients should I look for in a shampoo that will banish build-up?

A. Sodium laureth sulphate, which is a surfactant, adds cleaning properties to the shampoo – most shampoos have it. Avoid heavy conditioning shampoos which could add to the build-up problem. Good choices: Ion Clarifying Shampoo, Ion Balanced Cleansing Shampoo, Tresemme 4+4 Deep Cleansing Shampoo or Fantasia's 100% Pure Tea Shampoo.

7 Q. What shampoo should I use that will get rid of the mineral build-up caused by hard water?

A. Mineral build-up dulls hair's shine. A clarifying shampoo used periodically should help eliminate the build-up. Salon Care Ultra Moisturizing Anti-Chlorine Shampoo or Avec's All Pure Purifying Shampoo work well on all mineral deposits.

8 Q. What shampoo do I use to get rid of medications, such as antibiotics, in my hair?

A. Use a good clarifying shampoo like Ion Clarifying Shampoo or Avec's All Pure Shampoo.

9 Q. What makes a body-building shampoo work?

A. It cleanses without leaving any residual conditioner on hair. It has a rinse-clean factor to make hair feel fuller by leaving the cuticle slightly ruffled. Try Ion Balanced Cleansing, Jheri Redding Volumizer, or Biotera Revitalizing shampoos.

10 Q. My hair is straight, fine and very thin. Is there a particular shampoo that will give my hair body and fullness?

A. Try a volumizing formula, like Volumax, Jheri Redding Volumizer, Folicure or Professional Prescription Biotin Shampoo. The key ingredient is panthenol (Vitamin B-5) which acts to "plump up" the hair shaft.

11 Q. What are the benefits of natural sources, such as botanicals, eggs, honey, aloe vera, etc... in shampoo?

A. Natural source botanicals add proteins and conditioning agents to shampoo. They may be derived from plant and vegetable extracts or other sources. The benefit to hair is that they are proteins and moisture in a natural state. Biotera, Jheri Redding Professional Prescription Transpose and Aura shampoos contain natural extracts.

12 Q. I like to use botanical products on my hair. Do they clean my hair as well as other types of shampoos?

A. Many do clean just as well, since they usually contain a detergent which is needed for cleansing. Pure botanical extracts from flowers and plant oils can be found in Aura shampoos which are mildly refreshing, yet thoroughly cleanse hair.

13 Q. I would like to enhance my own natural hair color. What highlighting shampoos are available, and what do they do?

A. These shampoos have color added in the form of vegetable dyes that tone the hair. They are made to highlight or add depth to hair color, or provide a specific shading effect. Read the labels to find out what shampoo will enhance your hair. For example, choose Aura Shampoo with Madder Root for redheads, Clove for brunettes, Camomile for blonds, Black Malva for black hair, and Clairol's Shimmer Lights Gold Formula to add gold to blond hair. Also, Naturonics Jewel Tones Color Enhancing Shampoos come in four shades–from Black Opal, Tiger Eye (Brown), Red Ruby and Blonde Sapphire.

14 Q. I have gray hair which tends to look brassy. How do I take the yellow out?

A. You need to use a highlighting shampoo which contains vegetable dyes that tone down hair. These shampoos can minimize that brassy, yellow look with a gentle cool blue or violet base color. Try using Clairol's Shimmer Lights Original Formula or Jheri Redding Silver Lustre.

15 Q. My gray hair turned blue when I used a highlighting shampoo. What went wrong, and what can I use to keep it from looking brassy?

A. Gray hair can have many different textures and porosities which react differently to the amount of coloring found in toning samples. This is more of a problem with shampoos for toning brassiness on blond hair than for gray. Jheri Redding Silver Lustre and Aura Blue Malva have less blueing and are less likely to turn hair blue.

16 Q. Because I am allergic to detergents, what is a quality hypo-allergenic shampoo?

A. Look for a shampoo with natural ingredients, such as Aura or Biotera. If you are allergic to plants or natural extracts, you may have an allergic reaction. There is not a professional shampoo that is specifically hypo-allergenic or non-allergenic for all people.

17 Q. What shampoo is best for color-treated or permed hair?

A. Shampoos that are designed to control color loss are lower in pH, ranging from 2.5 to 4, which forces the cuticle of the hair to close, thus enabling the hair to retain its color. Try Quantum Shampoo for Permed and Color-Treated Hair, Keragenics Rejuvenating Shampoo or Preference After Color Shampoo by L'Oreal.

18 Q. My hair is really fried from perming. What type of shampoo will bring it back to life?

A. Normalizing shampoos take conditioning one step further. They are designed to revitalize hair dried out by chemical processes like perming. Sometimes they are called "perm rejuvenating" shampoos. Select a shampoo for permed hair, such as Quantum Shampoo for Permed and Color-Treated Hair, or Zotos Acclaim Plus Daily Conditioning Shampoo, Professional Prescription Transpose or Ion Moisturizing Shampoo.

19 Q. **What shampoo with sunscreen should I use to protect my color from fading?**

A. Try Aura and Biotera shampoos, as well as Professional Prescription Shampoos which contain conditioners and sunscreens.

20 Q. **I have dry hair, what shampoo should I use?**

A. For dry hair, use a moisturizing shampoo which cleans and conditions. A moisturizing shampoo has a rinse-out conditioner mixed in to prevent loss of moisture by closing the cuticle, and it helps fight dryness caused by blow dryers, curling irons, heat rollers and sun. Good ones to try are Ion Moisturizing Shampoo, Professional Prescription Transpose Shampoo or Apple Pectin Moisturizing Shampoo.

21 Q. **I get oily, greasy-looking hair at the end of the day. What can I do to end the greasies?**

A. Use an oily-hair formula shampoo, such as Professional Prescription Absolute, which can be used daily, or Quantum Clarifying Shampoo and Clarifying Shampoo from Ion, which should only be used twice a week. You may want to avoid using daily rinse-out conditioners, although you still need to condition hair. Fantasia IC 100% Pure Tea Shampoo also removes excess hair oils. Tea works as an astringent.

22 **Q.** I have normal hair that has been chemically treated. What would be a gentle shampoo for me?

A. Use a daily shampoo with gentle cleansing properties, such as a moisturizing shampoo. Try Fermodyl Moisture Recovery, Keragenics Therapy or Zotos Acclaim Plus Daily Conditioning Shampoo.

23 **Q.** What is a good no-rinse shampoo that can be used when I can't take a shower or bath?

A. Try No-Rinse, a shampoo that you massage into your scalp and comb through. Let it dry. There is no need to rinse this shampoo out. It's great if you are bedridden or camping outdoors.

24 **Q.** It never fails! By the end of the day I notice dandruff flakes in my hair. What type of shampoo will help?

A. Try a dandruff shampoo like Medi Dan, Medi Dan Extra or Queen Helene Dandruff Shampoo. They have an added ingredient that acts as a mild abrasive to shake dandruff loose from the scalp and wash it away. They are designed to remove OILY DANDRUFF, not dry dandruff, which is typically caused by overuse of chemicals or styling aids. If dandruff is from dry scalp, you can use a dry scalp shampoo or moisturizing shampoo. Medi Dan Dry Scalp Shampoo and other moisturizing shampoos, such as Ion Moisturizing Shampoo and Keragenics Therapy, will add moisture to scalp and hair. No dandruff shampoo will cure a medical skin condition such as eczema or psoriasis. If you suspect this is the cause, consult your doctor or a dermatologist.

25 **Q.** **How often should I shampoo my hair if I have dandruff?**

A. It depends on what type of dandruff you have. Medi Dan Plus can be used everyday because it has a conditioning formula. Stronger treatments, like Medi Dan Extra, should not be used everyday because it can be drying. This shampoo is best for dandruff combined with oiliness and flaking.

26 **Q.** **I have oily hair, but my scalp is dry and flaky. What shampoo should I use?**

A. Medi Dan Dry Scalp Shampoo will help alleviate the problem by cleansing hair well and still treating the scalp with medication to remove flakiness. Also try Fantasia IC 100% Pure Tea Shampoo.

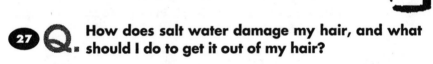

27 **Q.** **How does salt water damage my hair, and what should I do to get it out of my hair?**

A. When salt water dries on the hair, it creates a high-saline solution which can cause mineral deposits to build-up on hair, resulting in hair that is weighted down and cannot grow. Hair should be washed as soon as you get out of the water. MRX Swimmers Shampoo and Salon Care Ultra Moisturizing Anti-Chlorine Shampoo can remove salt water from hair.

28 Q. I have permed and colored hair and will be swimming in the ocean on my vacation. What shampoo should I use that will wash out the salt, yet not strip my color?

A. Consider Quantum Clarifying Shampoo or Salon Care Anti-Chlorine Swimmers Shampoo. Both will remove salt without damaging color-treated hair.

29 Q. What temperature should the water be when I rinse my hair after shampooing?

A. A cool water rinse helps close the cuticle, which makes the hair feel smoother. Hot water stimulates oil production, so if hair were dry, you may want to use warm water. If hair tends to get oily quickly, cool or tepid water is recommended. The temperature should be determined by what you want to achieve.

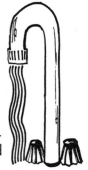

30 Q. How long should I rinse my hair after I shampoo?

A. The average time is 60-90 seconds. You know it is clean by the feel of your hair. Hair should not feel like it is coated. It is best to rinse hair with the water flowing in the direction of your cuticle, not against it – head is held back and water flows from forehead to back.

31 Q. How should I treat my hair after I shampoo it?

A. Blot, don't rub hair dry, as rubbing can cause tangling. Comb hair with a wide-tooth comb, holding sections of hair to gently comb through tangles.

SHAMPOO

_____

_____

_____

_____

_____

_____

_____

_____

_____

_____

_____

_____

_____

_____

_____

_____

_____

_____

SHAMPOO

_____

_____

_____

_____

_____

_____

_____

_____

_____

_____

_____

_____

_____

_____

_____

_____

_____

_____

_____

Treat Those Tresses

Imagine spreading a thick, greasy, gummy substance over your hair to condition it! That's what the ancient Egyptians did when they wanted to make their hair more manageable.

It was not uncommon to mix local fats and oils to create conditioners for the hair. One Egyptian solution consisted of a "mixture of six kinds of fat – the fat of a hippopotamus, a lion, a cat, a crocodile, a snake and an ibex."

Polynesians concocted a scented oil called "mouoi" and a gummy substance from the coconut tree called "pia" to create conditioners for the hair. The main problem with these early conditioners was they left the hair greasy, sticky and easily soiled.

It wasn't until the early 1950s that chemical suppliers realized the technology used in fabric softeners to soften natural wool fibers could also be used in creating conditioners for the hair. These early conditioners were emulsions that contained oils, such as mineral oils. They looked similar to cream hairdressings, but they could be rinsed out without removing the good properties of the conditioners.

From magical mixtures of wild animal fats, hair conditioners have progressed beyond the greasy concoctions of Cleopatra's day. Today, there are thousands of conditioners on the market, all claiming to solve specific hair problems, if not ALL of them.

F.Y. 👁

The Lowdown on Conditioners

Conditioners do a variety of things for your hair. Some work only on the cuticle and are used everyday. Others penetrate the cortex for longer lasting results. These are called deep-penetrating treatments, because they are used occasionally and are almost theraputic.

Deep-penetrating treatments are often packaged as single-application packettes or vials, because a little goes a long way! All open the cuticle to let moisture or protein into the cortex. Some treatments require heat: using a dryer, a heat cap or wrap. These are the most powerful conditioners.

There are two basic types of deep-penetrating treatments: moisturizing and protein. Moisturizing treatments put moisture, softness and "bounce" back into hair that's dried out from over-processing, heat styling or exposure to sun and wind. HOT OIL and CHOLESTEROL products are two types of moisturizing treatments, though there are others. Protein treatments may also be called "protein

We expect a lot from conditioners. They should add moisture, strengthen hair, make it shinier, detangle it, smooth split ends, add fullness and body, and more.

packs." They rebuild strength in hair that has lost its elasticity by adding protein to the cortex. Often this treatment is given before the perm or color to get hair into the best shape. Protein treatments are excellent when used as needed, but overuse can severely dry out hair.

Moisturizing and protecting are also attainable with daily conditioners, but they are not as strong as the deep-penetrating treatments. They are commonly called rinse-out or leave-in conditioners.

Conditioners work in a variety of ways, some only working on the cuticle and others actually penetrating into the cortex for longer lasting results. These latter conditioners are called deep-penetrating "treatments" because they are used occasionally for therapeutic reasons.

Conditioning and shampooing go together like salt and pepper. However, shampoos don't take the place of conditioning. Shampoos clean. Conditioners NOURISH.

32 Q. **I really like using a cream rinse. Is there a difference between a cream rinse and conditioner?**

A. A cream rinse detangles and doesn't penetrate like a conditioner will. They work instantly, but must be rinsed out well or they'll leave a residue, making hair look dull. A conditioner imparts moisture or protein to strengthen hair. Deep-penetrating conditioners actually penetrate the hair's cortex.

33 Q. Why do so many conditioners and styling aids contain alcohol? Doesn't it dry hair out?

A. The kind of alcohol found in some shampoos and conditioners is cetyl or stearyl alcohol. This type actually helps condition hair to make it softer. Isopropyl alcohol is in hairspray and some other styling aids, and is usually called SD-40 alcohol on the label. It is the ingredient which makes hairspray dry quickly. Generally, there is not enough SD-40 alcohol in any professional beauty product to be harmful. But remember, over time, they can build-up and sap hair's moisture. Shampoo well, and rinse thoroughly.

34 Q. My hair is really damaged. Will it help to leave in a conditioner longer than the directions indicate?

A. Not necessarily. Conditioners take a certain amount of time to penetrate the hair. After that time, there is no added benefit. Leaving conditioner in longer can actually do more harm than good by drying the hair out even more! Follow directions on the package or your stylist's advice.

F.Y. 👁

What is a humectant?

A humectant is an ingredient in hair products that draws moisture into the hair from the air. For dry hair, you want to be able to hold moisture. For fine, limp hair, you want to repel moisture.

35 Q. I have an oily scalp, but my hair is dry. What conditioner will treat those opposing conditions?

A. Use a gentle cleansing shampoo, then apply a rinse-out conditioner, like Ion Moisturizing Treatment or Professional Prescription Enforce, working the conditioner well into the ends. Rinse thoroughly.

36 Q. Why do some conditioners make your hair feel greasy?

A. That slick, oily feel can be a result of using too much conditioner, or applying a deep-penetrating treatment all over the hair, rather than just in spots that need it. Deep-penetrating moisturizing treatments should generally be used only on the damaged areas, such as dry or split ends.

37 Q. Is it important to use the same brand of shampoo and conditioner?

A. Yes, for best results, because as a system they are designed to work in harmony. However, it is not absolutely necessary.

38 Q. I think I have over-conditioned my hair. Help!

A. Over-moisturizing makes hair very limp. Hair that is over-proteined will be brittle and hard. Clarifying shampoos are the answer.

39 Q. What is a good everyday conditioner to use with an everyday shampoo?

A. Depending on the amount of conditioner needed, try Ion Finishing Rinse to make hair more manageable. Enforce by Professional Prescription offers more conditioning and can be used everyday. Unicure Hair and Skin Conditioner is a good everyday conditioner for simply detangling. For economy, try Salon Care All-Purpose Remoisturizer in the gallon size. Other great everyday conditioners are Zotos Acclaim Plus Daily Conditioner or Aura Rosemary & Mint Rinse.

40 Q. Which is best, a leave-in or rinse-out conditioner?

A. Rinse-out conditioners do more permanent conditioning by filling in the hair and making it stronger. Leave-in conditioners are made to maintain the hair on a daily basis. They make combing easier, which reduces friction, prevents breakage and adds sheen to the hair before drying. Leave-in conditioners also protect from additional moisture loss. Another leave-in conditioner, a perm rejuvenator, adds elasticity to the hair to encourage the curl pattern and add bounce. Moisturizers in the formula give the hair a healthy look.

41 Q. Can leave-in conditioners be used on all textures of hair?

A. Yes. On fine, thin hair, leave-in conditioners condition without weighing hair down. On coarse, thick hair, the conditioning agents will soften and make the hair easier to manage. Some good products to try are Keragenics Rejuvenating Treatment, Infusium 23, or Fantasia IC Hair and Scalp Treatment.

42 Q. I have fine hair. Should I avoid conditioners that weigh my hair down?

A. Conditioners of the past often seemed to plaster fine hair down on the head. Today, there are many lighter formulas. It may seem contrary to common sense, but a leave-in daily conditioner may actually work better for you than a rinse-out conditioner because it is formulated to be "lighter" on hair. Avoid conditioners that have waxy ingredients in them. Try using Jheri Redding Biotin, Volumizer Leave In or Zotos Acclaim Plus Leave-In Conditioner.

43 Q. Why should I use an instant conditioner after I shampoo?

A. To smooth the cuticle, making hair easy to comb. A smooth cuticle makes hair shine and look vibrant. Salon Care All Purpose Remoisturizer or Unicure Hair and Skin Conditioner both rinse out. Leave in conditioners include Ion Anti Frizz Leave In or Aphogee Pro Vitamin Leave In Treatment.

44 Q. Can leave-in conditioners be used everyday?

A. Leave-in conditioners are considered daily conditioners and can be used everyday. Try Jheri Redding Biotin, Biotera Leave In, Aura Elixer and Volumizer Leave In.

45 Q. I have oily hair. Should I use a conditioner?

A. Yes. It is best, however, to avoid using the rinse-out conditioners. A leave-in conditioner or deep-penetrating treatment may be needed, especially if hair is permed or color treated. Even oily hair can benefit from occasional moisturizing or protein treatments.

46 **Q.** **If I use a moisturizing shampoo, should I use a conditioner?**

A. In general, yes. There is not much benefit to following a moisturizing shampoo with a rinse-out conditioner – that's two doses of the same medicine! A leave-in conditioner, however, can complement a moisturizing shampoo, and there are many products designed to be used together in just this way.

47 **Q.** **What should I put on my hair before I wet comb it, after shampooing, so I will not break my hair?**

A. Use leave-in treatments such as Jheri Redding Volumizer Leave In, Infusium 23, Ion Anti Frizz Leave In, or Biotin Leave In Treatment for hair that needs extra nourishing and that is thin, fine or weak.

48 **Q.** **I have static in my hair. What can I do?**

A. Look for a product that will give a slight coating to the hair. Try a spray-on, leave-in conditioner. Most conditioners will help reduce static. Good products to try include Influx CHP Vitamin Treatment, Keragenics Rejuvenating Treatment, Aura Elixer or Ion Anti Frizz Leave In Conditioner.

49 Q. **My hair tangles easily. What will take out the tangles, but not weigh down my thin hair?**

A. Leave-in conditioners like Jheri Redding Volumizer, Ion Anti Frizz Leave In Conditioner, and Infusium 23 are light formulas that will not weigh hair down. Also consider using Keragenics Revitalizing Hair Treatment because it has panthenol and will help to re-moisturize hair.

50 Q. **I want to control my frizzy, fly-away hair. What can I use?**

A. Frizzy hair is often caused by dryness. Use a light moisturizer after every shampoo. Quantum Extra Care End Mend is good or try Ion Anti Frizz Leave In or Keragenics Rejuvenating Treatment. Frizzies caused by humidity are generally a result of having very fine, porous hair which causes the hair to swell in humid conditions. A solution to this problem is to use a light leave-in conditioner, like Ion Anti Frizz Leave In, which puts moisture in the hair. Also try Ion Anti Frizz Gel Mist, which is a styling product that controls curls and retains styles on the muggiest of days.

51 Q. **Is a protein treatment the same as a conditioner?**

A. Yes. Some conditioners work only on the hair's cuticle. These can be used everyday. Protein treatments rebuild strength in hair that has lost its elasticity by adding protein to the cortex, allowing hair to be strong and retain moisture. These deep-penetrating treatments often come in single applications, in packets or vials.

52 Q. Can a protein treatment be used on all textures of hair?

A. Yes, however to be most effective, protein treatments should be used on damaged hair. Healthy, coarse hair is already strong, and may only need extra moisture.

53 Q. How many times should you use a protein treatment?

A. It depends on the hair damage. If a protein treatment is used too often, the hair can become dried out. As a general rule, it is safe to use a treatment weekly for the first month to get hair in good shape. Then, use one or two times a month after that. Always follow the directions on the package or consult your stylist.

54 Q. A stylist told me that constantly pulling back my hair in a ponytail or using hot rollers too much can put me at risk for hair loss. What should I use to build strength and resilience?

A. First, be sure you are using protected hair bands to help minimize hair breakage. Don't pull hair too tightly or use hot rollers too often. Strengthen hair by periodically using protein treatments, such as Jheri Redding Natural Protein, Aphogee Protein Packs, Pantresse Vitamin Treatment Pack, or Keragenics Revitalizing Protein Packs. All add tensile strength to keep hair from breaking.

55 Q. The last time I got a perm, my hair was extreme-ly brittle afterwards. What can I use BEFORE I get my next perm to avoid this problem?

A. Use a protein treatment at least three times a week and a moisturizing conditioner after you shampoo on the other days prior to perming. A daily moisturizing treatment such as Quantum Extra Care Daily Moisturizing Treatment or Ion Moisturizing Treatment should help. For protein, try Ion Reconstructor, Fantasia IC Reconstructor or Jheri Redding Natural Protein Treatment.

56 Q. How often should I use a deep-penetrating treat-ment?

A. Use it once or twice a week, depending on the damage to your hair. Try it once a week for a month until hair is healthy. Then use the treatment once or twice a month there-after. Over-use can be harmful to hair and dry it out.

57 Q. When using a deep-penetrat-ing treatment, why should I cover or wrap my head?

A. Keeping the head warm helps open the cuticle layer and allows the conditioner to penetrate more effectively. The head can be wrapped with a hot towel or even in cellophane, like Glad Wrap! For easy, no mess cover-ups, try plastic processing caps like your stylist uses.

58 Q. I never have time for deep-penetrating treatments. When is best, morning or night?

A. It doesn't matter. You can, and should, condition anytime. If you want a deep-penetrating treatment, you may want to shampoo at night and condition while showering, wearing a plastic cap on the head so the conditioner penetrates better. If it is a conditioner that dries in the hair, you could do this at night and re-wet hair to style it in the morning. A daily, leave-in conditioner is a great answer to protecting hair from daily abuse of sun, wind and hot styling appliances.

59 Q. Should you shampoo after using a deep-penetrating treatment to remove residue?

A. No. You would be counteracting the conditioning process. All shampoos contain lauryl sulfate which removes oil from the hair.

60 Q. I am going skiing this winter. When should I have a deep-penetrating hair treatment?

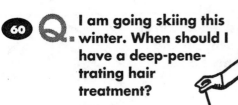

A. Conditioning should be planned monthly to protect hair. Cold weather has negative effects on hair due to the dryness. So, before winter sets in, condition to prevent problems.

61 Q. When I am under a lot of stress, my hair looks stressed out too! What type of treatment will revitalize my hair?

A. If hair is stressed because of over-processing, you need a deep-penetrating protein treatment. If hair is simply dry, a deep-penetrating moisturizing treatment, such as Ion Moisturizing Treatment, Ion Effective Care Treatment or Quantum Extra Care Weekly Hair Repair should be used. For everyday, try Keragenics Rejuvenating Treatment because it contains panthenol and is effective on all hair types.

62 Q. My hair is damaged from over-processing. What conditioner will put moisture and bounce back into my hair?

A. Most hair damaged by over-processing needs a combination of moisture and protein. The protein packs are excellent. Use a deep-penetrating protein treatment, such as Keragenics Revitalizing Protein Pack, Ion Effective Care & Intensive Therapy Conditioner Protein Pack and Aphogee Reconstructor Pack. For only dry hair, use a deep-penetrating moisturizing treatment. For hair breakage, try a deep-penetrating protein treatment. If it is dry and brittle, it probably needs a strong moisturizing treatment left on for at least 15 minutes. On a day-to-day basis, use a leave-in conditioner to protect hair, which seals the cuticle and keeps hair from being damaged further as it is brushed, combed or styled.

63 Q. When is the best time to apply a conditioner to the hair after hair has been colored?

A. Immediately after coloring (after shampooing). Use a conditioner which is formulated for use on color-treated hair like Wella In Depth Conditioner, Roux Mendex, Keragenics Revitalizing Pac or Fermodyl Treatment Vial Special Formula.

64 Q. My scalp itches in the winter. What conditioner can I use to relieve the itching?

A. Try a hot oil treatment which will moisturize the scalp and remove that itchy feeling, such as Keragenics Hot Oil. Aura Rosemary & Mint Rinse contains peppermint which soothes and cools itchy scalp.

65 Q. Can a person with thin, flyaway hair use a hot oil treatment?

A. Yes, but the results will be minimal because hot oil treatments are topical and can weigh hair down. Fine hair needs a protein treatment to build strength.

66 Q. Does a no-heat activated conditioner work as well as a heat activated conditioner?

A. It depends on what you are trying to achieve. For damaged hair, a heat activated conditioner may be more effective because heat tends to swell the cuticle so the conditioner penetrates the hair more readily. Ion Microwave Treatment, Ion Hot Oil, Let's Jam Hot Creme Treatment, L'Oreal Oleocap Lusterizer, Salon Care Cholesterol and Tresemme 4+4 Hot Oil are excellent options.

67 Q. What is the difference between a conditioner and a reconstructor?

A. A conditioner is often designed to add shine and manageability. The term "reconstructor" is used when the product has a high protein content to help strengthen hair. Examples of reconstructors are Aphogee Conditioning Treatment and Jheri Redding Keratin Reconstructor.

68 Q. My hair is thin and fine. Do I need a hair texturizer or hair thickener?

A. Both would work well, but differently. A texturizer styling lotion, such as Natural Balance Texturizing Setting Lotion, adds body and fullness and works well on most hair types. A thickener adds diameter to the hair by swelling the hair shaft. A good one to try is Fantasia Thick N'Hair.

69 Q. Because my hair is so thin, I continually have split ends. Is there something I can put on my hair to keep the ends from appearing split?

A. Condition and trim hair on a regular basis. Minimize the use of excess heat on hair with blow dryers, hot rollers and curling irons. Use a thermal styling lotion like Quantum The-mal Protectant before blow drying, or using hot rollers. For instant results, try a hair shiner which is a silicone based product. Rub shiner onto ends of hair and style. Shiners not only close the cuticle, but fill in gaps where it is broken. They won't solve the problem, but they make hair look shinier and softer! Try Ion Anti Frizz Hair Glosser, Replenishing Hair Shiner by Jheri Redding Professional Prescription or ACV Gloze. Be sure to follow directions. A tiny bit is all you need!

70 Q. When should I use a hair rinse or lemon rinse instead of conditioner? Will a vinegar rinse work as well?

A. Hair texture is the key. On fine hair, a lemon or vinegar rinse leaves hair with less tangles, but it could be too acidic for some fragile hair. Ion Finishing Rinse or Aura Rosemary & Mint Rinse offers the proper acid balance without the softening effect of a conditioner. Conditioners work best on hair that needs softening and manageability.

71 Q. Is there such a thing as a "mask" for your hair?

A. Yes, however, mud packs provide only temporary topical help. Try Naturonics Organic Mud Treatment, available in individual packs and an 8 oz. size. It is formulated with vitamins, minerals and botanical extracts to help restore moisture content and improve elasticity.

72 Q. I have hard tap water which dulls my hair. What can I do to improve the luster of my hair?

A. Minerals in hard water, like calcium and iron, bond to hair's protein making it dry and dull. Try Quantum Clarifying Gel Crystal Treatment to remove hard water build-up.

73 Q. What medications affect the condition of my hair?

A. Most all do. Medications are excreted through the hair, leaving a fine, thin film on hair. Quantum Clarifying Gel Treatment is designed to remove chemical traces from hair and is available in individual packets. It may also be used before a perm or chemical service in order for them to take properly. Consider also trying a clarifying shampoo.

74 Q. Does soft water affect the condition of my hair?

A. The salt used in water softeners can cause a build-up over time. Remove with a clarifying shampoo or treatment periodically.

C O N D I T I O N E R S

_____

_____

_____

_____

_____

_____

_____

_____

_____

_____

_____

_____

_____

_____

_____

_____

_____

_____

_____

Spritz, Sprays, Shiners 'N Gels

oday's styling products are a far cry from 1500 B.C. when the Assyrians first began styling hair as a profession. The Assyrians were so obsessed with hair styling that they were known throughout the Middle East for their expert skills in cutting, curling and dyeing the hair.

Not surprisingly, the Greeks of the Homeric Period believed that elaborate and complex hair styles denoted culture and distinguished them from the northern barbarians.

Fair hair was preferred, and perhaps one of the earliest styling products was a talc consisting of yellow flour and fine gold dust which was used to lighten the hair. Dusting hair in various colored powders was the height of fashion in 16th Century France. By the 1790s, the court of Marie Antoinette made powdering and all types of hairdressings the rage. Hair was combed, curled, waved, and piled high with false hair into towers that were then powdered in a myriad of colors.

Powder has gone the way of the guillotine, only to be replaced by the most high-tech of styling products that can shape, mold, wave, scrunch, curl and hold hair through the strongest of gale force winds.

There are gels, glazes, mousses, spritzes, sprays, shiners, stylers and waxes to create any look imaginable. And credit goes to the hairdresser, in most cases, who often conceived these products with an eye to the creativity and flexibility they provide.

75 Q. What is the difference between mousse, liquid, lotion, spritz, spray gel, glaze and gel?

A. Mousse is a light-hold, fast drying foam. Use on wet or dry hair. Mousse adds lift and fullness and can protect against heat and dryness. Liquids and lotions are medium-hold products worked through wet hair with the hands. They add volume, shape or style, control curls and define spiked styles. Spritz and spray gels are pump sprays usually used on dry or damp hair to sculpt or control it. They add body and texture. Spritzes tend to be stiffer than spray gels. Spritzing the base of hair helps it stand up from the roots and appear fuller. Spray gels can achieve the wet look. Glazes and gels are thick liquids used on wet or dry hair. Use for sculpting wet looks, for accenting particular curls or for controlling thick, wavy hair.

76 Q. I have very fine, thin hair, but my hair needs a lift! What type of styling product should I use?

A. Mousses work best for adding fullness and giving hair a lift. By applying it to the scalp, it can produce more fullness when damp hair is blown dry. Try using Jheri Redding Volumizer Mousse, Volumax Mousse, Ion Alcohol-Free Mousse or Aura Lemon Grass Mousse. A firm-hold hairspray will help keep fine hair in place.

77 Q. Is it better to use mousse or gel to style your hair, and when do you apply them, before or after blow drying?

A. A mousse or gel should be applied to the hair before blow drying. Most have an ingredient that helps protect the hair from the heat of the blow dryer. When applying a mousse or gel after blow drying, re-wet the hair to build extra body. Be aware, however, that you may not end up with the desired result because the hair may get weighed down or flattened if you apply these styling aids after blow drying. Good products to try are Jheri Redding Volumizer Mousse to add body, Ion Mousse for fine hair, Avec Mousse, Tresemme 4+4 Mousse and Stiff Stuff Volume Mousse. Spray gels are generally lighter formulations and tend to work better on fine hair because the spray allows for more even distribution. Try Volumizer Spray Gel. Thicker styling gels like Jheri Redding Styling Gel, Ion Anti Frizz Styling Gel and Salon Care Aloe Styling Gel are best used when doing a complete set or when working on the entire head. They also add body to the ends of hair.

78 Q. Gels thicken up and make my hair look dull. What can I use that will hold my hair, yet look soft?

A. Mousse is probably your best bet. It is the lightest-hold, yet most versatile styling aid. Use on wet or dry hair, overall, to fluff up and add volume, or apply it only to the sides of hair for a slicked-back look. You can also apply it just to the roots to make hair stand away from the head and appear fuller. Mousse is easy to use and combines some of the hold of a gel, with a softer, more natural feel.

79 Q. I would like to try a mousse to add body to my thin hair. How much should I use for short hair, medium-length hair or long hair?

A. For short hair, use a golf ball-size puff of mousse. For shoulder-length hair, fill the palm with mousse. For long hair, cover the palm and fingers with the mousse.

80 Q. I want to add body to my hair, but don't want a perm. What should I do?

A. Try having hair cut in layers and using a mousse or gel to give your hair body.

81 Q. Can you use a mousse on your hair if you have already used a conditioner?

A. Yes, you can use a mousse because it is a styling product. For light support, try Hair Specific Sheer Support or Ion Alcohol-Free Styling Mousse. For more support, try Volumizer Mousse or Tresemme 4+4 Mousse.

82 Q. Which styling product is least drying – a mousse or gel?

A. Gels tend to have more water which makes them less drying. Mousses sometimes have more alcohol, which can make them more drying. Consider using Ion Alcohol-Free Mousse or Jheri Redding Professional Prescription Alcohol-Free Styling Gel. Fantasia Liquid Mousse is also alcohol-free and contains panthenol for a healthy, shiny look.

83 Q. How can I revive my style at the end of the day?

A. Either brush through dry hair or retouch it with a damp comb, then spray again with hairspray. A spray gel works better than a mousse. If you already have gel in your hair and want to revive your style, try spraying on a leave-in conditioner to reactivate the gel, then restyle hair. Leave-in treatments include Ion Anti Frizz, Keragenics Leave In or Biotera Leave In.

84 Q. What is the best way to apply gel to hair?

A. Work the gel into the roots of the hair, which results in fullness and body. If you apply gel from the roots through to the ends, you can weigh the hair down. Apply gel first to the hands, rubbing gel on palms and fingers, then applying to the roots of the hair from the underside.

85 Q. I have a problem restyling my hair after I've gelled it. My hair is so stiff, it pulls when I brush it. What should I do to avoid hair breakage?

A. You may be using too much gel or a product that is too strong. The problem could also be that the product is not evenly distributed throughout your hair. Try using a glaze instead of a gel. You could also try using a leave-in conditioner before adding gel to the hair to provide more manageability, making it easier to comb hair after it dries.

86 Q. I love the natural look. How do I finger sculpt or scrunch curls in my straight or permed hair? What product is best to use?

A. Generally, a gel, spray gel or gel mist-type product works best for finger sculpting. To achieve this look, simply spray gel all over head, or work a regular gel evenly throughout hair. Lift curls at the base and continue lifting as the hair dries. Lifting is important because the moisture in the hair can weigh it down. What you are trying to do is lift the curl formation closer to the roots which achieves that "scrunched" look.

87 Q. What product can I use near my part, when I blow dry my hair, to add more volume at the crown?

A. Blow dry hair until it is completely dry. Then re-spray the part area with a root-lifting product, such as Quantum Root Lift, or use a spray styling gel at the root where hair parts.

88 Q. How do I get a really wavy look without a perm?

A. A wavy look requires a curl formation where the base of the curl is directed in alternating directions. For example, one row of curls is directed to the right, the next row to the left. Styling gels hold waves that are combed into short hair. Wave clamps work well to hold the waves in place until hair dries.

89 Q. What styling aid do I use to achieve the wet look?

A. Spray gels, glaze or gels achieve this wet look. Try Tresemme 4+4 Glaze, Professional Prescription Gel, Queen Helene Styling Gel, Biotera Gel or Volumax Glaze.

90 Q. I love the extra hold that gels offer, but hate the stiff, dull finish. What should I use that is light, yet leaves shine in my hair?

A. Use gels that are clear to give hair better shine. Use less of a gel product, or add water to the gel to reduce the stiffness. Good ones to try are Professional Prescription Styling Gel and Hair Fixative by JheriRedding, Salon Care Aloe Vera Styling Gel and Tresemme 4+4 Styling Gel.

91 Q. What is a styling glaze, and how should it be used?

A. Styling glaze is a firm-hold styling product that should be distributed evenly through hair. Use instead of a styling gel or other setting product. Try Volumax Glaze, Tresemme 4+4 Styling Glaze or Biotera Styling Glaze.

92 Q. I have flyaway hair, but love the look of "finger" or "molded" waves. Is there any hope for me?

A. Yes! Styling aids such as gels and glazes will help control flyaway hair. Also, hair shiners can keep those stray hairs under control. Try Ion Design Sculpting Lotion, Tresemme 4+4 Styling Glaze or Aura Constyler for finger or molded waves. Anti Frizz Gloss will help keep flyaway hair from becoming such a headache.

93 Q. What is a thermal styling lotion, and when should it be used?

A. Thermal lotions are specifically formulated with special ingredients that coat and protect hair from blow dryer and hot roller damage. Use a product like Quantum Thermal Protectant or Fantasia Ultra High Heat Styling Mist before blow drying or rolling with hot curlers. Leave-in conditioners like Fantasia IC Hair & Scalp Treatment or Keragenics Rejuvenating Treatment work well also.

94 Q. I set my hair everyday on hot rollers. Is there a styling aid that I should use to protect my hair?

A. Thermal styling lotions are designed to be used with styling appliances like hot rollers. Consider also using a spray gel for a crisper set or a mousse for a softer set. Styling products made especially for rollers and hot rollers include L'Oreal's Wave Chic and Stiff Stuff Roller Juice.

95 Q. What are setting lotions, and how are they used?

A. Setting lotions are medium-hold products designed to be worked through wet hair with the hands. They add volume, shape and style, control curls or define "spiked" styles. Good ones to try are Resque Ultimate Styling and Sculpting Lotion and Natural Balance Setting and Texturizing Lotion.

96 Q. My hair looks dull. What can I do to create more shine?

A. Hair shiners that spray on, rub on or are worked through the hair contain silicone or cyclomethicone, which coats the hair shaft to reflect light and add shine. They can be used before or after hairspray, but preferably before. Good ones to try are Aphogee Gloss Therapy, ACV Gloze Therapy Gloss, Ion Anti Frizz Glosser and Professional Prescription Replenishing Hairshiner. Spray-on formulas include Hask Pure Shine and Frizz Care. The key is to use shiners VERY SPARINGLY! A little dab does it!

97 Q. Is the silicone in my hair shiner harmful?

A. No. Most hair shiners contain water-soluable silicone. This is good for people with dull hair or split ends or if you want dramatic improvements fast. Silicone closes the hair cuticle and fills in gaps where it is broken. Try Volumizer Spray-On Shine, Frizz Care or Aphogee Gloss Therapy.

98 Q. Should a shiner be applied on wet or dry hair?

A. Hair can be dry or slightly damp. If you are doing a French braid, you want hair slightly damp. If hair will be in a style that moves, shiner should be applied on dry hair as a finishing product.

99 Q. Should shiners be applied on the hair or at the roots?

A. Generally, they are used to add shine to the hair, and thus, should be applied on the hair strand itself.

100 Q. I've been using a shiner, but it makes my hair look greasy. What is best for fine, thin hair, and how can I prevent that greasy look?

A. The amount of shiner you use varies with the amount of hair you have and its texture. For medium-length hair, use about the size of a dime, applied to the middle of the hand. Rub on hands first, then in hair. Try a spray-on shiner like Volumizer Spray-On Shine, Hask Pure Shine, Frizz Care and Let's Jam Oil Free Shiner.

101 Q. What can I use to control my hair when I French braid it?

A. Try silicone shiners such as Ion Anti Frizz Glosser, Professional Prescription Replenishing Hair Shiner or Frizz Care Hair Treatment to hold hair together and keep loose ends from flying. When hair is braided wet, apply a gel first, then a secondary application of a hair shiner. If hair is braided when dry, silicone shiners work well.

102 Q. What type of shiner is best for short hair?

A. Use a shiner in spray form because it will provide more even distribution.

103 Q. What type of shiner should be used on long hair?

A. Liquid shiners work best on long hair because you can distribute them through the hair with your hands, paying particular attention to dry, troubled areas, such as the ends or at the hair line. Try Jheri Redding Replenishing Hair Shiner, ACV Gloze and Wella Insta-Seal Recovery Treatment.

104 Q. I spritz my hair every morning, but it doesn't hold my set. What am I doing wrong?

A. It is easy to confuse spritz with hairspray, but there is an important difference. Spritz has holding resins like all styling support products. They add body and texture to a style. Hairsprays also have "memory" resins, which cause hair to "remember" the way it was styled and to return it to that style after it has been combed or fluffed. To hold a set, use a hairspray, like Grand Finale Hair Spray, Net Effect, Vita E and New Image Super Hold Hair Spray.

105 Q. Why does spritz make my hair look wet when I want a dry look?

A. A spritz or spray of any type should not make hair look wet unless it is being used too heavily or being sprayed too near hair. Spritz is a firm-hold and fast-drying spray that should be used SPARINGLY. Try Ion Super Hold Spritz, Tresemme 4+4 Styling Spritz or L'Oreal's Collection De Paris Spritz Finale for a dry look.

106 Q. Is there a hairspray you can wear everyday that won't coat your hair?

A. Some hairsprays are clean and tend to be less coating than others. A good example of this type of spray is Shaper Spray by the Generics Value Product, which contains a clear base and does not dull the hair. Also try Ion Hair Spray in the non-aerosol formula. Avoid freezing sprays because they contain more resin and are more difficult to get out of the hair. Spritzing sprays are designed to coat the hair to add body.

107 **Q.** **What hairspray won't make my hair flaky?**

A. Clear-formula liquid sprays generally go on smoothly and have less of a coating effect on the hair, and thus, tend to flake less. Flaking can also be caused by holding the spray too near the hair, resulting in a concentration of spray in one area. Ion Long-Lasting Liquid Hair Spray works well without flaking. If you prefer an aerosol, try Professional Prescription Ultra Control Hairspray or Vita E Hairspray. Both are clear aerosol formulas.

108 **Q.** **Is there a light hairspray that also offers super hold?**

A. The amount of hold provided by a hairspray is determined by the amount of resin in the product. Try Sheer Mist or Ion Hard to Hold hairspray.

109 **Q.** **Is there a difference between a "working" hairspray and a "freezing" hairspray?**

A. A working spray contains flexible resins that do not dry as firmly as the freezing-type resins. Freezing sprays are very firm holding and are designed to keep hair in a "fixed" position.

110 Q. I need a hairspray with ultimate hold. What will keep my hair in one place ALL day?

A. Products that offer ultimate hold are usually called freezing sprays. They are used for spot styling or problem areas or can be used all over on hard-to-hold hair. Check out Avec Instant Ultimate Hold, Jheri Redding Volumizer Freeze Spray or Volumax Freezing Spray.

111 Q. Will hairspray cause my hair to fall out?

A. There are no chemicals in hairsprays that will cause hair to fall out.

112 Q. My hair is chemically processed. What type of hairsprays should I avoid?

A. Generally, avoid sprays with a high amount of laquer or agents used for stiffening. These usually include freezing sprays. However, most hairsprays are water-soluable and are washed out of the hair.

113 Q. What hairspray can I use that will brush out easily?

A. Use a working type hairspray, such as Generics Shaper Spray, or Tresemme 4+4 Brush Out Shaping Spray. Due to their quick-drying formulas and light hold, these sprays brush out easily. Also AVEC Regular Hold and Aura Witch Hazel hairspray brush out easily.

114 Q. Which is better, a pump or aerosol spray?

A. Pump sprays go on wetter, and as a result, take longer to dry. Aerosols can provide more precise control for spot holding. It is really a matter of preference.

115 Q. Is it damaging to comb or brush hair that has been moussed or sprayed with hairspray?

A. Yes. Combing or brushing hair after applying styling aids can break and split hair. Wet hair first, then comb or brush before styling. Let hair dry. Then reapply the styling product. Avoid overuse of styling products if you comb or brush your hair often during the day. Be sure to use a wide-tooth comb or pick, or brush with flexible ball-tipped bristles.

116 Q. I hate build-up from styling products. Are there any that won't build up?

A. Most styling products are water-soluable. With proper use and regular shampooing, you can avoid build-up. It's probably a good idea to choose products from the same line because they are designed to work together, making it less likely they will build up.

117 **Q.** I noticed dandruff-like flakes after I started using a gel. Can I get dandruff from a styling product?

A. Not dandruff, but you can get flaking caused by an overuse of styling products. The best way to eliminate the problem is with proper shampooing. Use an everyday shampoo. Once a week or every two weeks, use a clarifying shampoo to get rid of any styling product build-up.

118 **Q.** What is the benefit of using styling products with sunscreen?

A. Styling products with sunscreens help protect hair from the sun's UV rays. As a result, they help keep hair from drying out or fading. Salon Care Quick Dry Sculpting Spray, and all Aura and Biotera styling products contain sunscreens. For prolonged exposure to the sun, consider more protection, such as sprays, mousses, even conditioners. Reapply after swimming to maintain protection.

119 **Q.** I have very thin hair, should I consider hair extensions?

A. Hair extensions are artificial hair pieces that are braided, sewn, woven or glued onto hair. They last about six months and should be tightened every month. Although hair extensions can be costly and time-consuming, the look may be well worth the effort. Always consult a trained professional for this service.

BEAUTY DIARY

SPRITZ, SPRAYS, SHINERS 'N GELS

_____
_____
_____
_____
_____
_____
_____
_____
_____
_____
_____
_____
_____
_____
_____
_____
_____
_____
_____

B E A U T Y   D I A R Y

SPRITZ, SPRAYS, SHINERS 'N GELS

_____

_____

_____

_____

_____

_____

_____

_____

_____

_____

_____

_____

_____

_____

_____

_____

_____

_____

_____

Tools Of The Trade

Where would the world be without a comb? Perhaps that question was asked more than 6,000 years ago when it is believed the first man-made combs were used by the ancient Egyptians. The most primitive comb is believed to be a large, dried fish backbone which is still used today by remote African tribes to groom and style the hair.

Because the comb resembles teeth, it is not surprising that the word "comb" is derived from the ancient Indo-European term, "gombhos," which means "teeth."

According to archeologists, with the exception of the Britons, all early cultures used combs. It was not until the Danes inhabited the British coastline in the mid-1800s that the Britons were taught how to groom their hair regularly with a comb.

Like the comb, the hair pin has a history that goes back hundreds of years. This seemingly simple styling tool was used by the ancient Greeks and Romans, not to mention Cleopatra, who preferred her hair pins in ivory and studded with jewels. In fact, the hair pin served a deathly dual purpose. Some were hollowed out to conceal poison, and it is believed that a hair pin of this design was used by Cleopatra when she poisoned herself.

F.Y. 👁

Roller Rap

There are 10 basic types of rollers:
- Magnetic rollers are used for wet sets to add smooth curls and lots of body.
- Velcro rollers are used on damp or dry hair to create soft curls and full-bodied styles.
- Foam cushion rollers are best for fragile hair and for sleeping.
- Snap-on rollers, which are brush rollers encased in plastic that can be sterilized, are used to hold hair to prevent slipping.
- Snap-on magnetic rollers are also made for fragile hair because they are gentle to hair and scalp.
- Plastic mesh rollers create smooth, beautiful curls and promote quick drying.
- Steam rollers steam-in long-lasting curls.
- Wire mesh rollers, in which the metal wire heats up with the help of the blow dryer, creates crisp curls.
- Brush rollers are designed to hold hair securely in place.
- Hair twirlers or flex rods create soft, natural curls without pins or clips and provide a variety of styles. They are specifically designed to create a spiral curl effect.

Thankfully, today's modern hair styling tools are designed solely for the purposes of grooming and styling the hair. And, they have expanded much beyond the earliest combs and hair pins to the most sophisticated of implements.

Professional styling tools range from a multitude of brushes, combs, clamps, rollers and ratts, picks and pins. Their usage is limited only by your imagination!

120 Q. **When should hair brushes be washed, and when should they be tossed!**

A. Personal hair brushes should be washed on a routine basis, depending on the build-up of natural oils from the scalp and the use of styling products. Use a comb to remove hair and wash your synthetic bristle brushes in warm water with mild soap or try Ship-Shape Brush and Comb Cleaner. Shake out excess water and air dry. For natural boar bristle brushes, dip in warm water using a mild detergent. Don't soak the brush as it can harm the bristles and the wood handle. Swish in water quickly to remove build-up and let brush dry naturally.

121 Q. **What are those round balls on the bristles of my hair brush?**

A. The round balls are epoxy ball-tips. The brush is dipped into the epoxy which creates the tiny balls. They help the brush glide through the hair more easily and prevent abrasions to the scalp, breaking or pulling of the hair.

122 Q. What is a boar bristle brush?

A. A boar bristle brush is one in which the filament or bristle comes from the wild boar. Usually the bristle comes from India or China where the animals are raised for their hair. Often, manufacturers will reinforce the boar bristle with heat resistant nylon to help the bristles penetrate the hair. Professional quality brushes to try include Lookin Good 7-Row 100% Boar Bristle Wave Brush and Phillips Super Round 100% Boar Bristle Brush. Reinforced boar brushes include Spornette RPB Round Brushes and Jerome Alexander Pure Boar Round Brushes.

123 Q. What type of brush will make my hair shine?

A. Boar bristle brushes make hair shine because they help pick up and distribute the hair and scalp's natural oils along the hair shaft as well as pull dirt or dust particles off the hair. A good one to try is Spornette #25 Porcupine Boar Brush.

124 Q. I have flyaway hair. What is the best type of brush for eliminating static?

A. Try an Anti-Static or Static-Free Brush. This type of brush has been made by blending carbon into the plastic. Brushes made entirely of wood generally are more static-free than others. Good static-free brushes to try include Cricket Fast Flow Ultra Vent, Tunnel Vent and RPM Round Brushes, and Continental W-Back Vent and Tunnel Vent Brushes.

125 Q. What type of hair tool can be used to give me the same effect as a roller?

A. If you are looking for a non-electrical tool, try "The Tong" brush, a barrel-shaped brush with clip attached, designed to be used with a blow dryer. It is available in a variety of sizes to achieve many of the looks rollers provide and can be used on all hair lengths.

126 Q. I would like to set my hair with Velcro rollers, but don't have the time everyday to let the hair air dry. What is the best option for me?

A. A round brush or tong brush with a cool setting on a blow dryer would speed up drying time without damaging the hair.

127 Q. I have curly hair. What is the best brush for me?

A. Generally, curly hair should not be brushed unless you intend to straighten it. In this case, the best brush is a natural reinforced boar bristle brush, such as Spornette RPB Round Brush or Jerome Alexander Reinforced Boar Rounder.

128 **Q.** My hair is board-straight! What is the best brush for me?

A. Use a brush that is gentle to the hair to prevent damage. Brushes with cushion bases and ball-tip bristles are best. Available in a variety of sizes and shapes for short to long hair, these brushes include the Phillips Avant-Garde and the Curlmaster Paddle Brush. Ball-tipped vent brushes are recommended for blow dryer styling.

129 **Q.** What is the best brush for fine, thin hair?

A. Use a wide-spaced, ball-tipped bristle brush. This will prevent breakage and add lift and volume while blow drying. Try the Cricket Static-Free Brush, the Static-Free Fast-Flow Brush, the Ultra Tunnel Vent Brush or Continental Tunnel Vent Brush.

130 **Q.** What is the best brush for long hair?

A. Use a large cushion paddle brush like the Curlmaster Paddle Brush. This type brush provides a larger base on which to brush the hair, thus allowing for more hair to be brushed with each stroke. Large round brushes, like the Phillips Super Round, are excellent for adding waves and curls to long hair.

131 Q. **What is the best brush for short, cropped hair?**

A. Use any vent brush with wide-spaced plastic bristles with vents penetrating the body of the brush for air flow, cushion or small round brush. It depends on what you are most comfortable with and the style you are trying to achieve. Vent brushes are designed for quick drying.

132 Q. **What is the best brush for my children's hair?**

A. Children's hair and scalp need extra gentle treatment. Use a very soft bristle brush for children under age 2. Once a child's hair has grown in enough to cover the scalp or reaches the shoulder, use a mild bristle brush for brushing the hair. Ball-tipped brushes are also gentle on the scalp.

133 Q. **I am 60-plus and have gray hair. What brush is best for me?**

A. Gray hair is usually more coarse and difficult to style. A stiff bristle brush like the Continental WNR21 Oval Cushion Brush or Continental WNR 9000DT Vent Brush is recommended.

134 **Q.** I am using a wire brush. Could this cause split ends?

A. Wire brushes without either an epoxy ball-tip or rounded or tapered ends will tend to break the ends of the hair because the wire ends are rough and can catch and pull the hair. These types of brushes are also rougher on the scalp. Try using a wire brush with ball-tips or tapered ends, such as the Stance Fanci Multi-Colored Cushion Brush or the Continental Wire Cushion Brush.

135 **Q.** Should I share my brushes and combs?

A. Sharing brushes and combs is definitely not recommended for health and sanitation reasons.

136 **Q.** When should combs be used?

A. Combs are best used on damp, towel-dried hair for combing through tangles. Combs are also used for sectioning hair, and can also be used on dry, short hair to fix a hairstyle. Wide-toothed combs are best for detangling hair. Basic combs include the Starflight Styling Comb and Rattail Combs.

137 Q. What type of comb should be used on wet hair?

A. A detangling comb is best for wet hair. Try Mebco's small or large detangler. Two rows of teeth are positioned to create a detangling effect on the hair. This is a must for long hair. A brush should not be used on wet hair because it can damage it by pulling and breaking the hair.

138 Q. What kind of comb should be used for "teasing?"

A. Special combs with small, serrated teeth between the longer teeth are used as teasing combs. The smaller teeth on the teasing comb pack hair toward the roots to create fullness and volume in the hair. The best comb for teasing depends on the thickness of hair. For fine, thin hair, use a comb with tightly spaced teeth to achieve volume and lift, such as Mebco Touch Up or Mebco Little Tease Touch Up. For thicker, coarser hair, a comb with medium to wide-spaced teeth with serrated edges is most effective, such as Comare Mark V Comb, Mebco's The Tease or Mebco Handle Pik.

139 Q. What is the best way for me to tease my hair so I don't damage it?

A. Use either a fine, medium or wide-tooth comb with serrated edges for teasing. Use a narrow-width comb for fine hair, medium-width for medium hair and wide comb for thick hair. To tease hair, do not pull on the hair too tightly. Hold the hair lightly at the ends and gently tease the hair just above the root line. This will add the volume you need to achieve lift. Carefully pick the hair to finish the style. Hair can be teased everyday as long as you are gentle.

140 Q. What are picks used for?

A. Picks are used to lift hair for volume and body. They finish a style or build fullness into the style without pulling the curl out. Picks are also great detanglers when hair is wet. Try Mebco's small, medium or large picks.

141 Q. I'd like to try Velcro rollers, but don't want them to fall out of my hair. Will I need bobby pins?

A. To properly use Velcro rollers without bobby pins, first section hair and comb smooth. Press end of hair section gently to roller. Then, roll firmly toward scalp, being sure hair is smooth and even on roller. Press each side of roller against the head to secure. The tiny loops on the surface of the Velcro rollers grab hair and hold it in place.

142 Q. How can I remove Velcro rollers without tearing my hair out?

A. Hold roller by the sides and firmly unroll away from the head. Do not try to pull or slip roller out. Premier Velcro rollers have a single Velcro loop and are more gentle on hair. They cause less breakage and do not tangle as badly as some brands.

143 Q. How should I curl my hair on non-heat rollers when it is dry?

A. Spray hair with either a spritz or spray gel, such as Fantasia Ultra High Heat Styling Mist or L'Oreal Wave Chic, then roll hair on Velcro rollers and blow dry. Other types of non-heat rollers can be used, but they generally require sitting under a hair dryer or using a bonnet style hair dryer which can be attached to your blow dryer.

144 Q. What size roller do I use to get lots of curls if I am using non-heat rollers?

A. Use small diameter rollers - 1/2" size - or pin curls. Apply a firm styling lotion, such as Ion Sculpturing and Designing Lotion before setting hair.

145 Q. How do I get a smooth, yet full, look using non-heat rollers?

A. Use jumbo rollers, such as the 1 1/8" Jumbo Blue, the 1 1/2" Bouffant Red, or 2" Giant Purple Velcro rollers and blow dry hair. After hair is set, smooth on just a dab of hair shiner first before blow drying.

146 Q. My hair is coarse, curly and thick. What non-heat roller is best for me?

A. Use a roller that will allow air to flow through the hair to promote faster drying. Velcro or plastic mesh rollers would work well for you.

147 Q. How many different sizes and types of Velcro rollers are there?

A. Sally Beauty Supply carries two different Velcro rollers – the single and double loop styles. There are 12 different sizes.

148 Q. What are the best rollers to sleep in?

A. Velcro or Foam cushion rollers.

149 Q. I like using magnetic rollers. How do they differ from Velcro rollers?

A. Magnetic rollers are used for wet sets. Magnetics give a smoother and longer lasting curl because they are usually used on wetter hair. Velcro rollers are used primarily on dry or slightly damp hair to create soft curls or full-bodied styles.

150 Q. My hair is fine, thin and straight. What is the best non-heat roller for me?

A. Magnetic rollers are usually the best bet for fine, thin hair because they do not "grab" the hair and there is little chance of breaking the hair. Styling Essentials' magnetic rollers come in 13 different sizes to achieve any curl you want.

151 Q. What is the best way to hold my non-heat rollers in place?

A. Special wire roller pins or double prong roller clips.

152 Q. My hair is short and straight. How do I get wave and curl without a perm?

A. Use small diameter rollers or pin curls for a curly look, and wave clamps for waves. Use a firm styling lotion before setting hair. Blow dry hair with a diffuser and let cool before brushing.

153 Q. My hair falls flat after I set it on rollers, what's wrong?

A. You could be rolling your hair improperly or using a roller that is too large for the type of curl you want. To roll hair, hold the hair section at a 45-degree angle from where you part your hair, and roll hair directly back onto the base of the hair section. Secure roller.

154 Q. **My hair gets the frizzies from rollers. What happens?**

A. You could be setting your hair on rollers that are too small for the type of curl you are trying to achieve. Also, be sure that each hair strand is combed completely smooth before rolling it onto the roller.

155 Q. **After setting my hair on rollers, what is the best way to dry my hair for the most lasting curl?**

A. Using a hot dryer – either convertible bonnet or hard-bonnet type – will set the curl fastest and give the longest lasting curl. Remember to let curls cool before combing through or you'll weaken the curl formations. Same is true when using a curling iron.

156 Q. **I love the look of a French roll. My stylist suggested a ratt. What is it?**

A. Ratts are hair foundations used to create fullness and sophisticated hair rolls, like the French roll. They can be used on all types of hair, from extra-thick to extra-fine hair. Ratts are made from featherweight foam for comfort and durability. You can even sleep on them! To use a ratt, position the foundation on the hair where you want the roll. Fasten each end of the foundation to the hair with a bobby pin. Push the pin through the foundation or pin over the foundation by squeezing the end. Smooth hair over the foundation and tuck the ends of hair under the foundation with a comb or brush. Fasten with hair pins. Voila! French roll!

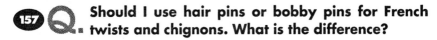

157 Q. Should I use hair pins or bobby pins for French twists and chignons. What is the difference?

A. Hair pins are open at the end and are used to hold large amounts of hair in place. Bobby pins are crimped at the end to hold small amounts of hair tightly. Both are used to create the base or support for either a French twist or to hold a chignon ratt in place.

158 Q. How do you set pin curls?

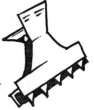

A. Twist hair, wrap around a finger, then clip in place; or tie two strands of hair together in several knots, then wrap around a finger and clip in place.

159 Q. What kind of clip should I use for pin curls?

A. Double or single prong clips.

160 Q. What can I use to hold my bridal headpiece in place?

A. Combs can be sewn into the headpiece, or use white hair pins or white bobby pins which will not show.

161 Q. What is a banana clip and how do I use it?

A. A banana clip is used to pull the hair back in a cascade style. It is used like a ponytail holder, but has combs that grip the hair and clips at the top. Many banana clips have pearls or ribbons attached and are used as a fashionable accessory.

162 Q. I want to do something special with my hair. My stylist suggested "hair jewelry." What is it?

A. Hair jewelry consists of hair beads, charms and gems that are glued or pinned onto the hair. A special hair bonding glue is used that washes easily out of the hair. Jewelry is used for hair decoration, and many up-do's feature it.

163 Q. What is the best hair accessory to pull my hair off the face without breaking my hair?

A. Use headbands or head wraps, stretchy cloth twisters or terry cloth ponytail holders. Consider also rubbing conditioner onto the covered elastic bands so bands will not break hair.

164 Q. I like to cut my own hair because it is long, straight and thick. What type of trimming shears are best?

A. A shear with one serrated edge, such as the Fromm Sharp Shear, helps to keep the hair in place while being cut rather than pushing the hair away.

165 Q. **I have split ends. How often should I have my hair trimmed?**

A. Every 4 to 6 weeks.

166 Q. **When should I use end papers on my hair?**

A. End papers are designed to use on hair that is being permed. End papers may also be used to protect fragile hair when it is being rolled on hot rollers, and are sometimes used on wet sets when hair is rolled on magnetic rollers. They are also helpful in controlling unruly hair that is being set on rollers, particularly when you don't want to risk over-use of gel to control stray ends. Tip: Fold paper over end of hair or place one at top of strand and one on bottom, at end of hair. Make sure hair is smooth. Then roll from end paper up.

B E A U T Y   D I A R Y

T O O L S   O F   T H E   T R A D E

_____

_____

_____

_____

_____

_____

_____

_____

_____

_____

_____

_____

_____

_____

_____

_____

_____

_____

_____

B E A U T Y   D I A R Y

T O O L S   O F   T H E   T R A D E

_____

_____

_____

_____

_____

_____

_____

_____

_____

_____

_____

_____

_____

_____

_____

_____

_____

_____

_____

_____

Plug It In

Thomas Edison made it all happen, for without him women around the world quite probably would still be relying on the sun's rays to dry their hair!

Even before electricity was harnessed, hair was styled with heated implements. As early as 1500 B.C., fire-heated iron bars were used by Assyrian slaves to curl the long tresses of kings, warriors and noblewomen.

The invention of electric hair dryers, blow dryers, curling irons, steam rollers, pressing combs, brushes and crimpers have revolutionized the way women style their hair today. Versatile, time-saving, packable, styling appliances owe much of their invention to two unrelated electrical appliances – the vacuum cleaner and the blender.

During the early 1920s, the idea of blow drying hair originated with vacuum cleaner advertisements proclaiming more than one use of the vacuum cleaner. By hooking a hose to the exhaust of the vacuum, one could easily dry her hair. The idea, however, had a catch. What was needed was a small motor to make the hand-held blow dryer a reality. An appliance that did have a small motor during this time was the electric milk shake mixer and blender, invented in Racine, Wisconsin. In effect, the exhaust of the vacuum was added to the small motor of the blender to produce the modern hair dryer.

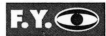

What's Hot

Today's most popular styling appliances are: the hand-held blow dryer, the curling iron, hot rollers, steam rollers, the flat iron or crimping iron, the hot air styling brush, and hair dryers, including the bonnet-type which can be attached to a blow dryer. Each do different things.

• Hand-held blow dryers are used to dry wet or damp hair, as well as to style the hair while drying. Blow dryers generally are used on high speed and hot settings if hair is very wet, otherwise, low speeds and warm settings are best. They range in power from 1250 watts to as high as 1700 watts.

• Curling irons create individual curls by rolling hair on an electrically heated barrel that varies in diameter from very small, 3/8" to jumbo size, 1 1/2". They are often used for touch-ups, spot curls, or all-over curls, and come in two basic types: the spring clamp which requires only the use of your thumb, or the Marcel iron which requires the use of the entire hand. The spring iron is much easier to use.

Over the next 30 years, the hair dryer was re-fined with the first major improvement in portable home hair dryers consisting of a hand-held dryer and plastic bonnet that connected to the blower and fit over the head. This $12.95 hair wonder was featured in the 1951 Fall/ Winter Sears cata-log. Ten years before, beauty legend Jheri Redding invented the first hooded hair dryers for use in hair salons.

Only recently have we seen such an explosion in hair appliance technology. In 1971, Conair was credited with introducing the first pistol-grip blow dryer to the United States, thus signaling the birth of shampoo-and-blow dry hair styles that revolu-tionized the way hairdressers and their clients style their hair.

Today, few women (and men) would want to be without their blow dryer, as evidenced now by the number of blow dryers which are standard equipment in most hotel bathrooms.

> • Hot rollers are heat-ed on a base. Each roller retains heat and as it cools, it sets the curl.Rollers come in small, medium and large diameters, and are used for spot curls or all-over. Hair should cool before brushing to avoid brushing out the curl.
>
> •Steam rollers are sponge rollers held in place by a clamp and heated by steam. As the steam cools, it evaporates and mois-turizes the hair. They give hair soft curls and waves which last longer than hot roller sets.
>
> • A flat iron or styling comb straightens curly hair. The very high heat set-ting is used for straightening and styling coarse, thick, curly hair.
>
> (continued next page)

 Q. **What is the difference between professional blow dryers and the "drugstore" variety?**

A. Professional blow dryers have more powerful, longer-lasting motors, which allow for greater air velocity and hotter tem-peratures. Some professional dryers do go up to 1700 watts, which is higher than most common varieties. Professional blow dryers are also made from a more durable plastic.

168 Q. **What is the proper way to blow dry hair?**

A. Hair should be slightly damp when you start blow drying. Use medium heat and high speed for most styling and setting procedures. Select lower heat and speeds for finishing hair styles. Lower heat and speeds should be used for drying and styling permed, color-treated or fragile hair. Whenever you brush hair and partly blow dry it against its natural growth pattern, you will add bulk and body to the style. After partially drying hair in this manner, then brush hair and blow dry it in the direction you want your finished style.

169 Q. **I travel overseas a lot. What can I do to make my blow dryer and hot curlers work on my trips?**

A. Use a current adaptor and find out what the current is where you will be staying. Curlmaster and Avanti both make travel dryers that are dual voltage for world-wide use.

• Crimping irons create a tight, wavy effect. Hair is divided into sections approximately 2 1/2" wide by 3/4" deep. The hair sections are placed between the hot crimping plates and clamped down firmly for two seconds. Hard-to-curl hair takes longer.

• Hot air styling brushes work like a blow dryer and curling iron combined in that warm air is forced through a vented barrel which has "teeth" that grabs the hair as it is curled around the brush. They are used on damp hair to give soft, light curls or wave.

• Hair dryers are used for wet sets, whether they are the salon variety you sit under, or bonnet-type that can be attached to your blow dryer. Salon dryers are designed to dry hair faster than the home bonnet variety.

170 Q. **What should I look for in a travel hair dryer?**

A. A travel dryer should be lightweight, have a handle which folds in for convenient storage, and have dual voltage for worldwide usage. It should have at least two speeds and two heat settings. Curlmaster's 1250 Watt Travel Dryer or Avanti's 1600 Watt Travel Dryer are excellent choices.

171 Q. **How close should I hold my blow dryer to my hair?**

A. Hold dryer eight to ten inches to remove moisture, and four to six inches from hair when styling.

172 Q. **How long should I dry my hair in rollers under a bonnet-type hair dryer? What setting is safest for hair?**

A. 20-45 minutes is usually sufficient for drying a roller set, depending on the length of your hair. The setting should never be so high you are uncomfortable or your scalp burns. It is always safest to dry hair on a lower setting for a longer period than to use a high setting for a short time. Switch to a cool setting for the last five minutes.

173 Q. My blow dryer sometimes turns off in the middle of drying. What could be wrong?

A. First, unplug the dryer and let it cool down. Check the intake vents on the dryer to be sure they are not clogged. You may also be holding the nozzle of the blow dryer too close to the hair. This will also cause the dryer to overheat. Reset the switch on the safety plug.

174 Q. When using a hair dryer, what heat setting should I use?

A. A hair dryer should be used on the warm setting most of the time. However, the hot setting should be used sparingly in short bursts when removing excess moisture just after hair has been towel dried. A hot setting never should be used directly at the roots or scalp. The cool setting should be used at the point at which the hair is dry. Cool air sets the hair in place.

175 Q. Should you dry your roots only and leave the rest of your hair slightly wet?

A. No. For best results, dry all of your hair, beginning at the root area and working out toward the end, otherwise, let your hair dry naturally.

176 Q. Do blow dryers damage hair?

A. No, not when used properly. Don't over dry hair. Use highest heat setting only when hair is very wet.

177 Q. What hair dryers are available that offer a low or cool setting?

A. Avanti 1600 Watt Turbo Dryer, Curlmaster Turbo 1600 with Cool Shot, Curlmaster 1600 Watt Dryer, Curlmaster 1250 Mid-Size Dryer, and Gold N' Hot Professional Hair Dryers in 1200, 1500 or 1700 wattages are some choices.

178 Q. What type of hair dryer is best for someone who does not like to spend a lot of time drying their hair?

A. Use a high wattage professional hair dryer since it outputs hotter air. Consider Avanti 1600W Turbo Dryer with Cool Shot, Curlmaster Turbo 1600 Watt Dryer, Yellowbird or Blackbird 1600 Watt Dryer, the Curlmaster Turbo 1600 Watt Dryer with Cool Shot Trigger, the Gold N' Hot 1700 Watt Dryer, or the Helen of Troy 1700 Watt Dryer with Cool Shot.

179 Q. What is the best type of hair dryer for thin hair?

A. A dryer with at least two air flow settings as well as various heat settings. For best results, use low air settings and medium heat.

180 Q. My stylist uses a heat lamp to dry my hair. What can I use at home to get the same effect?

A. A blow dryer with a diffuser attachment will achieve the same effect as a heat lamp.

181 Q. I have small hands. What blow dryer is best for me?

A. Many blow dryers have contoured handles designed for any size hand. Look for these handles on the box. Select a medium size, lightweight dryer, like the Curlmaster 1250 Watt Dryer.

182 Q. What should I look for when I buy a blow dryer for everyday use?

A. For everyday use, your blow dryer should have at least two speed settings and three heat settings. A removable grill for easy cleaning and an 8-ft. cord are important features, too.

183 Q. What are those nozzle attachments that came with my blow dryer?

A. The nozzle attachments are called "air concentrators." They direct the air flow to a smaller area, concentrating the air on one spot.

184 Q. What is a diffuser and how is it used?

A. A diffuser is an attachment which fits on the barrel of a blow dryer to disperse the air flow and spread it over a larger area. All diffusers should be used on low speed and cool to warm heat settings. Using a diffuser with a dryer set on high defeats its purpose and can cause the dryer to overheat. A flat-vented diffuser or "finger" diffuser can be used on naturally curly or permed hair styles. The diffuser dries the curl softly and slowly so the curl pattern is not disturbed. This type of diffuser is excellent for drying straight hair at the roots to add volume and lift. Simply bend at the waist and direct air flow at the nape of the neck and roots of the hair. Keep the dryer moving. Never let the air stay directed at the same spot for any length of time.

185 Q. Which is better, a diffuser with or without "fingers?"

A. Both are excellent for drying naturally curly or permed hair. A "finger" diffuser can be used to lift and separate the hair, adding volume while drying the hair. It is better for long hair. A flat-vented diffuser achieves the same result, except you need to lift and separate the hair with your free hand while keeping the diffuser in motion over the area being dried. Try the Curlmaster or Helen of Troy Euro Diffuser.

186 Q. What is an easy-to-pack, inexpensive diffuser?

A. Try the Soft Air Dryer Mit Diffuser or the Soft Diffuse-Aire Diffuser, which fit any hair dryer and are especially recommended for naturally curly, permed or wavy hair. Simply slip the dryer mit over the hand blow dryer nozzle and blow dry hair.

187 Q. Every time I use my hair dryer, I seem to blow away my style. What can I use that will pinpoint one specific area and dry it?

A. To blow style your hair without hot gusts of air dashing your style, attach the concentrator nozzle on your dryer and use the low speed setting to dry a specific area.

188 Q. Does drying hair under a convertible bonnet dryer take longer than a salon hair dryer?

A. A salon hair dryer is designed to output a higher air velocity which will dry the hair faster than a home bonnet dryer. Another option for home use is the portable "hard hat" dryer that resembles a salon dryer. Lady Carel's offers 1100 watts of drying power and the Gold N' Hot Hard Hat has 1200 watts.

189 Q. Are hoods for drying hair available as attachments for blow dryers?

A. Yes. There are vented bonnets with an attached hose which connects directly to the barrel of a blow dryer, such as Avanti's Soft Bonnet Dryer Attachment.

190 Q. Are curling irons available with different types of coatings? What is the best type to prevent damage to hair?

A. There are several different types of coatings. Chrome-plated irons are the most common and most popular, and can be used on all hair types. For thin, fine hair, use on low heat. For medium to coarse hair, use on high. Gold-plated barrels are used on irons which have higher heat capabilities. They are best used on medium to coarse hair. The curling irons with non-stick coating are like Teflon cookware. These barrels are coated with a material which prevents the hair from sticking to the barrel, making them an excellent choice for fine to medium hair.

191 Q. What is the difference between a spring iron and a Marcel iron?

A. A spring iron has a spring mechanism on the clamp which brings it down and holds it tight to the barrel surface. A Marcel iron has a clamp which is controlled manually by the user, and is most often used by salon professionals. The spring iron is much easier to use because it requires only the use of your thumb to control it.

192 Q. What size and type curling iron is best to achieve a tight curl?

A. The shorter the hair, the smaller the barrel size needed for the tight curl. The barrel size should increase in relation to the length of hair, up to 3/4" barrel. Larger than that will not achieve a tight curl. Try the Helen of Troy or Curlmaster 1/2" spring curling iron.

193 Q. **What size and type curling iron is best to achieve a wave?**

A. For a wave, a larger barrel size is best. Depending on the length of hair, the 3/4" to 1 1/2" size will offer a nice wave. Try the 3/4" spring iron by Curlmaster, the 7/8" or 1" spring iron by Helen of Troy or the Grand Champion 3/4" or 1" spring iron.

194 Q. **Which is more damaging to the hair, a curling iron or electric rollers?**

A. Neither, when used properly. Always follow the manufacturer's instructions.

195 Q. **If your hair is not completely dry when you use a curling iron, will it burn your hair?**

A. A curling iron should only be used on completely dry hair because the steam created from excess moisture and the heat from the iron can cause scalp burns. Never use a hot curling iron at roots or scalp.

196 Q. **I have naturally curly hair that is always out of control. Is there a curling iron available that will straighten my hair without leaving it frizzy?**

A. A large-barrel, professional curling iron that reaches a higher temperature will work better on curly or frizzy hair. Try a 1" barrel for light curl or a larger 1 1/2" or 1 1/4" for super smooth hair. The Gold N'Hot Curling Irons have a rheostat temperature control ranging from 145 to 320 degrees.

197 Q. How soon can I use my hot rollers or curling iron after a perm?

A. This depends on your hair type and the perm used. Technically, they can be used immediately after hair is dry. For fine or fragile hair, wait 24-48 hours.

198 Q. What is the difference between a hot-air styling brush and a curling iron?

A. A hot-air styling brush works like a blow dryer. Warm air is forced through a vented barrel which has "teeth" to grab and curl the hair while style drying. Use only on damp hair to finish styling the hair. Hot-air styling brushes give soft, light curls or waves. A curling iron does not dry hair like the hot-air styling brush can, but it does give hair a tight curl. Curlmaster makes a hot-air brush in 1/2" or 3/4" sizes.

199 Q. Is chrome or Teflon better for a curling iron?

A. It depends on your hair type, although both are equally suited to most hair types, from thin and fine, to medium and coarse hair.

200 Q. I have gray, thinning hair. Should I use hot rollers or a curling iron?

A. For everyday, a curling iron with low heat setting would be your best bet. For curls or waves with added volume, try a steam hair setter which will set hair without drying it out. Good choices include Curlmaster Dual Heat Curling Irons, Belson Profiles Steam Express Hairsetter or Caruso Molecular Hairsetter.

201 Q. How should I clean my curling iron?

A. First, unplug the iron and let it cool down. Use a soft, slightly damp cloth to wipe the surface. Do not allow water or any other liquid to get into the unit. Use a non-abrasive cleaner on the chrome barrel, and baking soda on the Teflon type.

202 Q. What can I use instead of electric rollers to achieve a quick set?

A. A curling iron is a good, quick alternative.

203 Q. What is the best size curling iron to use on bangs to curl them back?

A. Either a 5/8" or 3/4" barrel size will be the most effective. They are available by Curlmaster, Grand Champion or Helen of Troy.

204 **Q.** What is a flat iron and how is it used?

A. A flat iron or straightening iron, such as the Gold N' Hot Straightening Iron, is used to straighten hair.

205 **Q.** How many different brands of flat irons are there?

A. There are four or five different brands. Belson makes the Gold N' Hot Professional Straightening Iron, #9087.

206 **Q.** I have naturally curly, thick blond hair and look like Shirley Temple. What can I use to straighten it?

A. Use an extra-large barrel curling iron if hair is short, or a flat iron such as the Gold N' Hot Straightening Iron.

207 Q. I have extremely coarse, thick, curly hair. I would like to straighten my hair without using a flat iron. What can I use?

A. Try a styling comb, such as Belson's Gold N' Hot Precision Styling Comb. It has been specially designed to straighten or style very coarse, thick hair.
Its variable temperature heat controls provide very high heat for straightening and styling thick, coarse hair, and very low heat for styling extra fine, damaged or dry hair, as well as a full range of heat settings for all normal textures and thicknesses of hair.

208 Q. I like that tight, wavy look, but I don't want to get a perm. What styling appliance should I use?

A. Try a crimping iron like the Gold N' Hot Crimping Iron. To crimp hair, work with hair sections that are about 2 1/2" wide by 3/4" deep. Place a hair section between the hot crimping plates of the iron and clamp down firmly. Hold in place for only a few seconds. Easy-to-curl hair will take about two seconds to crimp. Hard-to-curl hair will take a little longer. Continue until all sections have been crimped. Hair can be picked out for fullness.

209 Q. What is the difference between steam rollers and hot rollers?

A. Steam rollers use moisture to lock in curls, while hot rollers use dry heat.

210 Q. Are steam rollers better for your hair than electric hot rollers?

A. Hair set with steam rollers will last longer than a style set with hot rollers due to the moisture cooling off the steam rollers. As the moisture cools and evaporates, the curl is set. Two good options are the Caruso Molecular Hairsetter or Belson Profiles Steam Express Hair Setter.

211 Q. Is there a benefit to using steam rollers?

A. The benefit in using steam rollers comes from the moisture from the steam. As the steam cools, it evaporates and moisturizes the hair, leaving the hair soft and shiny. The set from steam rollers gives the hair soft curls and waves which tend to last longer than curls from hot rollers.

212 Q. Will electric rollers damage my hair?

A. Not when used properly. Always read and follow the manufacturer's use and care instructions on any appliance. Be sure to let the electric roller cool down before removing rollers so that the curl sets. Removing the curlers before they cool can cause hair to frizz. The new foam cushioned steam rollers with smooth plastic clamps are the most gentle to hair.

213 Q. What type of hot rollers should be used on thin, flyaway hair? How do I keep them in the hair?

A. Steam rollers are best for thin, flyaway hair. They are easier to use on thin hair because the hair is held in place on the sponge roller by a clamp which covers the entire curl. Try Belson Profiles Steam Express Hair Setter or the Caruso Molecular Hairsetter. Try using the 2-3 inch wide butterfly clamps on your electric rollers if they slip out.

214 Q. What is the most practical set of hot rollers for someone with short hair?

A. For short hair, look for a set that has more small and medium size rollers such as the Belson Profiles Deluxe Hairsetter with 24 rollers. The hot rollers with raised nobs will grip hair best.

215 Q. I have layered hair that is board-straight. What is the most practical set of hot rollers for me?

A. Any good professional hair roller set that gets extra hot, such as the Belson Profiles Hairsetter which comes with 18 or 24 rollers.

216 Q. I have hair, dirt, dust and spray build-up on my hot rollers. How can I clean them?

A. Soak the curlers in hot, soapy water, then scrub them with a small brush. Rinse and allow them to dry thoroughly before putting them back on the heating unit.

217 Q. How long should hot rollers heat up before using them?

A. Most hot rollers have either a "ready dot" on the individual rollers themselves or an indicator light that goes on when rollers are ready to use. Hot rollers are heated on posts which are designed to heat up to a maximum temperature, and then to maintain that level. Rollers should not be left on more than 45 minutes.

218 Q. What direction should I roll my hair on hot rollers?

A. Roll the hair in the direction you want the curl. Rolling the hair over the top of the roller will curl the hair up. Rolling the hair under the roller will make a pageboy style. If the hair is styled back, roll away from the face, if hair is styled forward, roll toward the face.

219 **Q.** I have a small bathroom and the electrical outlet is above the sink. I'm afraid of dropping my appliances in the sink and shocking myself. Are there appliances that have electric shock protectors?

A. There are many styling appliances that have automatic shut-off functions in case they are accidentally immersed in water. Most professional dryers have this feature, i.e. Curlmaster 1250 Watt Dryer, Gold N' Hot 1700 Watt Dryer, Conair Avanti 1600 Watt Turbo Dryer and Helen of Troy 1500 Watt Dryer with Cold Shot.

220 **Q.** Where can I get my hot rollers and blow dryers repaired?

A. Contact the manufacturer of the product for their repair. If the item is under warranty, return it to the manufacturer; otherwise, contact the manufacturer to see if they offer repair services or can refer you to someone in your area.

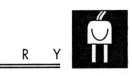

BEAUTY DIARY

PLUG IT IN

_____

_____

_____

_____

_____

_____

_____

_____

_____

_____

_____

_____

_____

_____

_____

_____

_____

_____

_____

_____

_____

Curl Talk

Not everyone was born with curls, but to look back in history at the artifacts, sculptures and masterpiece paintings, one might think otherwise.

Throughout time, curls have been valued for their status, their religious significance, their political message and their sheer appeal.

Men and women have endured the unthinkable simply to have a crown of curls atop their head. Ancient Egyptians heated irons to curl royal beards and wigs. The Greeks used irons and terra cotta rollers. In Rome, the wealthy curled their hair on hollow tubes that were heated by inserting a hot rod. During the Renaissance, "crisping irons" were introduced at the Italian Court. All kinds of curling contraptions were used to create temporary curls.

It was not until the early 20th Century that a man named Marcel became famous for his way of waving hair in Paris. But it was Charles Nestle who is credited with creating the first permanent wave machine in London in 1905. Nestle's machine involved winding the hair in a spiral on a rod, coating it with an alkaline paste and covering all with an asbestos tube and a heated gas pipe-size iron with tong handles. Electricity was used to heat the large iron clamps while hair was held in place until it had been sufficiently steamed. This method was called croquignole wrapping, used primarily

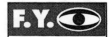

What makes a perm work ?

Hair is made of keratin, composed of long molecular chains within the cortex layer of hair. These chains form a twisted rope-like fiber which has a network of cross-bonds or links that provide stability, strength and elasticity to hair. There are two types of bonds: hydrogen bonds and cystine or sulphur bonds. Permanent waves change the hair from straight to wavy by breaking these cross-bonds. When hair takes on its new shape, the bonds must be re-established for curl to be permanent.

The classic permanent wave solution or "cold wave" lotion is generally thioglycolic acid plus ammonia, which causes the cystine or sulphur bonds to be released. When hair is wrapped on the rod, this solution is applied. A certain amount of time is required for the hair to take on the shape and size of the rod. This is called "processing time." Once the hair is "processed," the stylist applies a neutralizer while hair is still on the rods. The neutralizer provides a dual chemical action, neutralizing and oxidizing, which results in reforming the cystine bonds and the hydrogen bonds so that the hair stays curled. The neutralizer forms new hydrogen bonds to shrink or harden the cortex and cuticle layers of the hair. The cystine bonds are reformed by oxidation that occurs between the sulphur in the hair and the active oxygen atoms in the neutralizer. When the cystine bonds are reformed, the wave remains permanent. After all the neutralizer penetrates the hair, hair is unwrapped carefully and rinsed thoroughly with water. Now, hair is ready to style.

For best results, perms should be done by a salon professional.

on short hair. The entire perm took at least six hours, after which the clients got plenty of curl, and often frizzy, dry, damaged hair with it!

Thankfully, a machineless perm was born in the 1930s, called a "cold wave," now also called an "alkaline wave." In the 1940s, liquid neutralizer was introduced. When perms fell out of fashion in the 1960s because natural looks were "in," acid perms were developed to create softer curls. More recently, conditioners were added to perms to enhance the hair and improve its look.

Today's perms continue to offer many improvements, and there are numerous perms that can be given at home. For best results, see your hair stylist for a professional perm. And, between salon visits, to maintain those glorious curls and wonderful waves, pamper your perm properly!

221 Q. **What is the difference between home permanents and professional permanents?**

A. Home perms are usually milder formulas that take longer to process. Professional perms have the advantage of the most current technology and an experienced stylist to help ensure the results.

222 Q. What is a cold wave?

A. The cold wave is an old term used for an alkaline wave. This type of perm does not require any added heat to process.

223 Q. What is an exothermic perm?

A. Exothermic perms contain ingredients that generate their own gentle heat and improve penetration of wave lotion.

224 Q. What is a bisulfate perm?

A. This is another form of chemical compound that has the potential to curl hair.

225 Q. What is a root perm?

A. Root perms are used at the root area of the hair only. They are used to perm new growth on the hair that has been previously permed or to add extra lift at the root area. The previously-permed ends are protected with products to prevent the waving lotion from penetrating the ends.

226 Q. What is a reverse perm?

A. A reverse perm is actually the process of taking curl OUT of hair. It can be used to change a naturally tight curl to a looser curl. It is often referred to as straightening hair.

227 Q. What is a spiral perm? What is the difference between this type of perm and a traditional salon perm?

A. A spiral perm means that shoulder-length or longer hair is rolled onto the perm rod vertically, resulting in a corkscrew-type curl. Spiral perms can also be used to create an explosion of curls. For a traditional perm, hair is rolled horizontally.

228 Q. My stylist suggested I try a weave perm. What is it?

A. A weave perm waves only part of the hair to provide fullness and curves rather than curl. It is not an easy perm to do, so be sure your stylist is skilled.

229 Q. Is there a perm on the market that is chemical-free?

A. No. A perm must have chemicals, whether natural or synthetic, in it to break the disulfide bonds in the hair and then rearrange them into the new, desired curl pattern.

230 Q. My new perm is too curly. What can I do to relax it a little?

A. First, condition hair immediately, then blow-dry hair using a large brush. You may also need to set hair on large rollers. Never use chemical straighteners or relaxers for permed hair because they could damage it.

231 Q. How tight should you pull perm rollers if you want a curly look versus waves? Does it matter how tight the perm rollers are rolled?

A. Tension is not a factor to consider when deciding between curly or wavy patterns. Rod size, wrapping techniques and the perm formula chosen determine whether you have curly or wavy hair. Most manufacturers recommend wrapping with minimal tension to avoid damage to the hair. Let your stylist know if you feel the perm rods are wrapped so tight that they are uncomfortable.

232 Q. What causes a perm to be frizzy?

A. Usually, it is caused by using too much tension when wrapping a perm. Minimal tension should be used so the cuticle can open freely to receive the perm solution. It is important for your stylist to follow directions carefully.

233 Q. I hate my new perm. Can I get it redone immediately?

A. Go back to your stylist and discuss the alternatives. If it is too curly, it can be relaxed. If it is not curly enough, wait at least a week to redo it. If your hair is not in good enough condition to re-perm, you may have to trim your hair and wait until your hair is ready to perm again.

234 Q. I need something to revive my perm. It's only a few weeks old, and it has gone limp. What can I do?

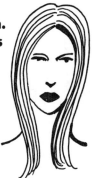

A. Perm rejuvenators contain moisturizers that add snap to a curl. Avoid heavy conditioners that could weigh hair down. Consult your stylist before the next perm and suggest a different type perm, change of rod size or wrapping technique. Try Quantam Perm Rejuvenator or Design Freedom Perm Revitalizer.

235 Q. My last perm lasted less than a month. What went wrong?

A. There are numerous reasons: a bad choice of perm or formula; too much water used during wrapping; not enough water blotted from hair before neutralizing; the stylist missed or skipped a step; hair had excess build-up; a poor consultation in which the client forgot to tell the stylist something that could have affected the way the perm reacted; too much or too heavy conditioning during your daily regime could also cause curl to relax. Discuss your problem with your stylist.

236 Q. I'm three months pregnant, and my last perm was five months ago. My hair is a wreck! Can I have it permed now?

A. Consult your doctor first. Generally, it is safe for a pregnant woman to perm her hair, as long as she doesn't drink the solution! Many stylists recommend waiting until after the first trimester.

237 Q. I like the look of a pageboy, but my fine, thin hair droops by the end of the day. What perm will give me this sleek look that lasts?

A. Body waves are perfect for this look because they'll provide the curve and volume you need to hold your pageboy style.

238 Q. My hair is in that awful growing-out stage. What can I do to survive this period?

A. Let your stylist trim or cut your hair. He or she may also use a spot perm on the new growth. The hair also can be permed on the undersections of the hair to give shape and to make the growing out less noticeable.

239 Q. Can I safely have my hair colored and permed?

A. Yes, if your stylist uses the correct perm and follows all procedures correctly, and your hair is in good condition at the time of the service. Let your stylist be your guide.

240 Q. Will a perm change my haircolor?

A. A perm should not change your natural haircolor. Many perms do fade color-treated hair. Your stylist should rinse hair thoroughly to remove all perm solution from hair to prevent any color fading.

241 Q. Why is it important for me to consult with my stylist before I have a perm?

A. All perms are designed to be used on specific hair types. It is important for your stylist to consult with you first to determine exactly what you want from a perm. It is also important for the stylist to know your life style, medical conditions or time limitations to select the right formula. Then, the stylist must choose the correct wrapping technique and rod size to achieve the results you desire.

242 Q. How long before a wedding should a bride-to-be have a perm?

A. One to two weeks so that the stylist can create a look the bride knows she will be happy with immediately.

243 Q. How often is too often to perm my hair?

A. The normal time period between perms is three to four months as long as hair is trimmed or cut two or three times within this period. Your stylist can help you make this decision.

244 Q. The last perm I had lasted six months. What did my stylist do to make it last so long?

A. Your stylist chose the correct perm and rod size and correctly performed each step of the perming process.

245 Q. I swim daily in an indoor pool for exercise. Can I have my hair permed?

A. Yes. Hair should be classified as "chemically damaged" because it has been exposed to a high level of alkalinity everyday. Your stylist will select a perm for you based on this. Be sure to shampoo after swimming with a swimmer's shampoo like Salon Care Anti Chlorine Moisturizing Shampoo.

246 Q. Should I have my hair cut before or after a perm?

A. Consult with your stylist. Some stylists prefer to cut hair before the perm to remove excess length and weight. Others prefer to cut after the perm to remove any dry or damaged ends and to shape the style.

247 Q. How do I know my hair is in good enough condition to perm?

A. Your stylist will check to see that you have good elasticity and enough moisture in your hair.

248 Q. My hair is thin, dry and flyaway. Can I have it permed without damaging my hair?

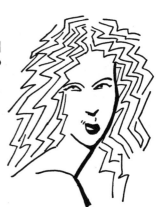

A. Consult your stylist. Your hair will need extra moisture before perming. A deep moisturizing treatment may be applied to your hair prior to the perm service.

249 Q. Can I go bald from perms?

A. Perms do not cause baldness. Hair, however, can break off if too much tension is used during the wrapping technique. Also, if the rubber band on the perm rod is twisted, hair can be broken off at the scalp.

250 Q. I get the "greasies" easily. Can I wash my hair after my perm?

A. If you shampoo immediately after perming, you can relax the curl. Wait at least 48 hours before washing your hair. Until then, wear a hat or pull hair back with a pretty hair accessory.

251 Q. Can I use a blow dryer right after my perm?

A. You can, but it is best to use a low setting and a diffuser. If you brush the hair while drying and pull it straight, you risk relaxing the curl.

252 Q. Can I use gel or mousse on my hair immediately after a perm?

A. Yes. A lighter spray-on gel works great on permed hair. Try Aura Flax Seed Spray-on Gel (flax acts to seal cuticle), L'Oreal's Dynamic Curls or Hair Specifics Spray Light Gel. An alcohol-free mousse like Quantum or Jheri Redding Volumizer won't dry out curls.

253 Q. How should I treat my hair after I shampoo my new perm?

A. Gently blot excess water from your hair. Then spray with a leave-in treatment like Great Feeling Curl Revitalizer or Ion Anti-Frizz Leave-in because they won't weigh curls down. Avoid pulling or picking the hair until it is almost dry to avoid breakage and the frizzies.

254 Q. What medications affect the results of a perm? Should I tell my stylist what medicines I am taking?

A. Yes, always tell your stylist what medications you are taking, and if you have had any recent surgery, including cosmetic or reconstructive surgery. Because medications are excreted through the hair, they could possibly affect the outcome of a perm. Among the types of medications that effect perm results are hormones and high blood pressure medications which tend to make a perm "take" faster than normal. It is believed that these medications raise the temperature of the scalp which accelerates the perm process. Low blood sugar medication can cause early curl relaxation. Retin A can cause the scalp to be more sensitive to chemicals resulting in a burning sensation. Iron supplements can cause the hair to be more resistant to perming. Ask your doctor what effect specific medications may have. It is also a good idea to use a clarifying shampoo before a perm.

255 Q. I work in the sun on weekends. My permed hair is beginning to look parched. What should I do?

A. If at all possible, wear a hat. Also, use styling products with sunscreens, such as Aura and Biotera. Use a daily shampoo and conditioner that will add moisture to the hair.

256 Q. Do botanical perms differ from chemical perms? Will they last as long?

A. All perms contain chemicals in order to work. Botanical perms differ from other types of perms in that they have added botanicals and herbs. Yes, they do last as long!

257 Q. What can I do to get rid of that yucky perm odor in my hair?

A. There are products available that can be used immediately after a perm to remove residual perm odor. Your stylist should be aware of them. Be sure your stylist rinses your hair longer the next time you have a perm to ensure that all the waving lotion is removed. Many new perms are being introduced that have a more appealing smell. If you are particularly sensitive to perm odor, tell your stylist before having the perm service.

258 Q. Can I have a cold wave perm every three months?

A. Yes, it depends on your hair texture and hair styles. Some short cuts will require frequent perming.

259 Q. I had a soft wave at home. When can I have my hair re-permed?

A. If hair is in good condition, you can re-perm immediately if you want more curl. However, it is best to consult your stylist.

260 Q. How can I cut down on the time I am at the salon for a perm, yet be sure my hair is properly conditioned before the perm service?

A. Your stylist can use a leave-in conditioner on the hair with some of the new perm products which not only saves you salon time, but also leaves your hair in excellent condition after the perm. Consult your stylist about using this procedure.

261 Q. What is the best size perm rod to get the tightest curl?

A. The smaller the rod size, the tighter the curl. However, perm formulas provide various strengths and snap to curl. Show your stylist a picture of the style you want so he or she can determine the best rod size to use.

262 Q. What is the best size perm rod to achieve waves?

A. Your stylist will probably use a larger rod size. For very little curl and mostly waves, suggest your stylist use the largest perm rods available.

263 Q. I have fine, medium-texture hair. What is the best perm for me?

A. Your stylist may use a cold wave, or a more gentle formulation such as the acid-balanced perm which is heat-activated. This type of perm usually results in soft, loose waves without the risk of frizzies.

264 Q. I want a perm that allows me to wash, dry and go. What type of perm should I request from my stylist?

A. Your stylist may recommend a curly perm. For best results, your hair should be cut in longer, graduated layers, rather than short layers all over, otherwise you could look like a poodle! The cut is critical.

265 Q. My hair is damaged by sun and chlorine. What perm should my stylist use?

A. First, you should use a clarifying shampoo to remove the chlorine build-up. Then, consult your stylist regarding whether your hair can be permed. If the sun lightened your hair, a perm for color-treated hair should be used. Your hair may also need moisturizing treatments or conditioning before the perm service.

266 Q. What type of perm should I get for my hair when it is growing out from a perm?

A. A perm specifically designed for dry or damaged hair would be your best bet. Let your stylist be the guide. He or she may also want to use a moisturizing pre-wrap on your hair to add extra moisture to the dry or damaged areas.

267 Q. My hair falls in my eyes constantly. What perm would help this?

A. Your stylist would use a directional wrap that forces the hair away from the face and into the desired direction. If your hair is very heavy, you may want to use styling aids to keep the hair in place after you style it.

268 Q. I only want height at the crown. What perm is best for this?

A. Your stylist would use a spot or root perm.

269 Q. I am of Asian descent with coarse, straight hair. What perm should I have?

A. Any coarse hair can be permed. Coarse hair is hard to wrap, but not hard to perm. Your stylist would probably use a cold wave and take extra care in wrapping your hair.

270 Q. What conditioning program should I use before my perm?

A. You should not need a specific conditioning program before perming unless your hair is severely damaged. In this case, consult your stylist.

271 Q. What kind of hairspray can I use on my new perm?

A. Consider using a working spray that will easily rinse out or brush out, such as Tresemme 4 + 4 Brush Out Shaping Spray or Ion Hair Spray.

272 Q. I live on the Gulf Coast, and it is so humid my perm frizzes. What can I do?

A. Use a styling aid to hold hair in place and to seal the cuticle. Use products that contain special humectants and other ingredients to help control the frizzies, such as Ion Anti Frizz Glosser or Frizz Care Hair Treatment.

273 Q. After a perm, my hair always looks dull and lighter than its original color. What can I do?

A. Make sure your stylist is thoroughly rinsing the perm solution from your hair, because applying a neutralizer over the perm solution can cause dryness and lighten haircolor. Consider using a shiner on hair, or a color-enhancing shampoo, such as Aura, which corresponds to your natural haircolor.

274 Q. I love to ski, but when I am in the mountains my permed hair "dies." What can I do to rev it back up?

A. Try a perm rejuvenator like Quantum, Great Feeling or Design Freedom Perm Revitalizer to perk up your hair.

275 Q. What special products should I use after I perm my hair?

A. Permed hair may need extra conditioning. Try Quantum Shampoo and Conditioner for Permed or Color Treated Hair or Keragenics Rejuvenating Treatment and Shampoo.

276 Q. My hair is naturally very curly. What products and methods are available to straighten my curls?

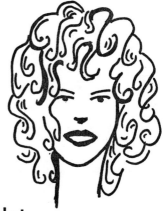

A. Certain wrapping techniques and extra large perm rods can soften curly hair. Chemical relaxers can also be used to straighten naturally curly hair.

277 Q. For a more natural look, what different types of perm rollers should my stylist use?

A. All perms should look natural. The choice of rod size and type should be discussed with your stylist before wrapping begins.

C U R L T A L K

_____

_____

_____

_____

_____

_____

_____

_____

_____

_____

_____

_____

_____

_____

_____

_____

_____

_____

_____

_____

_____

CURL TALK

_____

_____

_____

_____

_____

_____

_____

_____

_____

_____

_____

_____

_____

_____

_____

_____

_____

_____

_____

_____

_____

_____

_____

For Women Of Color

For centuries, African women have regarded their hair as an important reflection of their heritage, often decorating it grandly to reflect tribal or family customs.

Today, fashion trends, movies, celebrities, recording artists and sports figures set the direction for the way many African-American women style their hair, rather than customs passed down through the ages.

Because African-American hair is characteristically curlier and coarser than Caucasian hair, numerous hair care products have been developed over the years to specifically address the needs of black hair. One person, in particular, is credited with launching the modern black hair care revolution – Madame C. J. Walker. This orphaned daughter of Louisiana ex-slaves built a multi-million dollar hair care business from a single ointment she concocted on her stove in 1905.

"Madame Walker," as she was to become known, developed not only an influential beauty business, but also numerous hair care products including an innovative pressing comb.

Still in existence today, Madame Walker's company, along with other major ethnic product manufacturers, offer African-American women products specifically designed for their hair and skin. Some of these top companies include Soft Sheen, Luster's, Johnson's Products, Pro-line, Summit Labs and J M Products.

Thanks to these companies, women of color have hundreds of options available to help keep their hair healthy, shiny and beautiful. And best of all, these modern hair care products are quick, safe and easy to use!

278 **Q.** I'm interested in having my hair chemically straightened but I don't completely understand the process. Exactly what does relaxing involve?

A. When a woman's hair is relaxed, it is chemically straightened. A relaxer works by penetrating into the cortex and breaking the strong chemical bonds that made hair curly. Relaxing hair begins by protecting the skin around the scalp with a protective cream or oil. Then, a relaxer chemical is applied to dry hair a section at a time, and hair is processed for a specified time. Hair is then rinsed and a neutralizing shampoo is applied to stop the relaxing process. Because relaxing can leave hair in a weakened condition, a deep-penetrating treatment is often the final step. A mild straightening solution should be used on fine hair. Hair that is thicker and more coarse can take a stronger solution. For touch-ups, a relaxer is applied only to new growth about every six weeks. Relaxers are strong chemicals that are best used by your stylist.

279 **Q.** I hate the smell from relaxers. How can I minimize this unappealing odor?

A. Unfortunately, while your hair is being relaxed, you can't avoid the odor. However, after relaxing hair, shampooing well with a good neutralizing shampoo, like Sheenique or Isoplus Neutralizing Shampoo, will help remove the odor.

280 Q. If I have coarse hair, what would be the best relaxer for me?

A. A super strength is best for very coarse or resistant hair and preferably a sodium hydroxide relaxer. See your stylist for the best advice.

281 Q. What is the difference between regular, super and mild relaxer strengths?

A. The amount of active chemical (sodium hydroxide or calcium hydroxide) determines the strength of the relaxer. Regular is for most people with normal hair, super for very coarse or resistant hair and mild for fine.

282 Q. What is the difference between a relaxer and a curl?

A. A relaxer straightens the hair while a curl (also called a perm) re-forms a tight curl into a looser, more manageable curl.

283 Q. What is the difference between lye and no-lye relaxers?

A. The difference is in the type of chemicals used. In lye relaxers, the active ingredient is sodium hydroxide. In no-lye relaxers, the active ingredient is calcium hydroxide. The no-lye relaxer is usually a little milder and good for sensitive scalps, but the calcium can cause hair to be slightly drier.

284 Q. **My 10-year-old daughter wants her hair relaxed. Is she too young?**

A. Years ago, relaxers for children were not even thought about. In addition to being painful, chemical straighteners used to smell awful, were unpredictable, and carried a high risk of permanent hair and scalp damage. Today, relaxers are much gentler on the hair and scalp and can be controlled. In fact, several manufacturers make chemical straighteners just for children, such as Soft Sheen's Tender Care Relaxer Kit, Pro-line's Just For Me Relaxer Kit or Lustre's PCJ No-Lye Relaxer Kit. Many manufacturers recommend having a child's hair analyzed first.

285 Q. **How often can hair be relaxed?**

A. Just like permanent haircolor, new growth on hair that's been relaxed needs to be "touched up." This is usually done about every six weeks. The whole head should never be re-relaxed. Relaxing is tougher on the hair than any other chemical process, therefore, only "new growth" should be "touched up."

286 Q. I relaxed my hair, but as soon as I shampooed it, the curliness came right back. What happened?

A. The relaxing process may have been stopped too soon. When that happens, it can look like the hair is completely relaxed, but when it is rinsed and shampooed, the natural curl is still there! The process must be correctly timed. Look for instructions that might indicate how long you should wait to shampoo or consult your stylist.

287 Q. I have relaxed hair. What type of hair regime should I follow? For natural or thermally-styled hair? For curled hair?

A. For relaxed hair, shampoo once a week, and use a rinse-out conditioner as well as a leave-in conditioner twice a week. Use a hairdressing or oil sheen daily. For natural or thermally-styled hair, shampoo once a week, use a leave-in conditioner after shampooing and use a hairdressing or oil sheen daily. For curled hair, you shampoo every week to 10 days, then use a curl activator everyday and curl moisturizer about twice a week.

288 Q. Can you use a no-lye relaxer over one with lye?

A. Yes. Because the relaxer is always applied to new growth only, not over previously relaxed hair.

289 Q. Why is it necessary to use a neutralizing shampoo with a relaxer?

A. A neutralizing shampoo is used after a relaxer to help remove all traces of the relaxer and help return the hair to its normal pH level.

290 Q. Will moisturizing my hair cause my hair to go back to it's curly shape after it is relaxed?

A. No. Moisturizing is important to keep hair in tip-top shape – so don't be afraid to do it regularly, after every shampoo. Good moisturizing products to try are Ion Moisturizing Treatment, Queen Helene Cholesterol or New Era Hair Moisturizer.

291 Q. I don't want to completely straighten my hair. Is there a way to loosen the curl and add texture?

A. A texturizing relaxer or a mild relaxer combed through the hair and left for 19 to 20 minutes will loosen the curl. Kits made specifically for this include Pro-line's Comb Thru Texturizer, Luster's S-Curl Kit or Sportin' Waves Comb-Thru Kit.

292 Q. Does a relaxer curl or straighten hair? What is the difference?

A. A relaxer is designed to straighten hair. A curl product first relaxes hair, then a waving lotion or booster is used to curl hair. After curling, hair is neutralized like a standard perm would be.

293 Q. Can African-Americans use any type of perm product?

A. Yes, depending on their hair type. Chemically, a curl product and a conventional alkaline permanent wave have the same active ingredient: ammonium thioglycolate. The difference is that most curl services call for that first "loosening" application of thio (the "rearranger") before applying the waving lotion.

294 Q. Can relaxed hair be chemically curled? Can curled hair be relaxed?

A. No, not at the same time. The two processes are different, and the chemicals are incompatible with each other. To do both would break the hair and cause severe damage.

295 Q. What is the safest way to grow out a curly perm?

A. Continue to keep your hair maintained with curl maintenance products. Wash and condition regularly and moisturize the new growth. For maintenance, try Care Free Curl Hair & Scalp Spray, Wave Nouveau Finishing Mist and Lotion or Right On Curl Activator Moisturizer.

296 Q. Is there a way to curl my hair without using chemicals?

A. Try roller setting with a body building product such as Lottabody Setting Lotion, or Ultra Sheen Super Setting Lotion. They'll provide protection and a firmer curl, too!

297 Q. Can I color my relaxed (or curled) hair?

A. Sure you can! But double-processing is tough on any hair and double-processing relaxed hair can be especially dangerous. The best recommendation is usually not permanent haircolor. Use semi-permanent color instead, or use an "in-between" type color, which doesn't have any lightening action, but can last almost as long as permanent haircolor. It is best to consult a professional stylist for coloring relaxed or chemically curled hair.

298 Q. Can I use henna on my hair?

A. Regular henna is not recommended for use on hair that has been chemically treated. Ardell's Hennalucent is a 100 percent organictranslucent toner and conditioner that can be use on permed or relaxed hair safely. In fact, it will restore elasticity, body and shine as it contains hydrolyzed animal protein, plant extracts and henna.

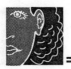

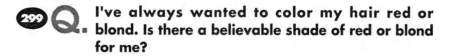

299 **Q.** I've always wanted to color my hair red or blond. Is there a believable shade of red or blond for me?

A. There is a shade of red or blond for everyone! The key is knowing whether you should go red or opt for blond. Ask yourself what hue your hair turns in the summer? Does it have a red or blond cast? Use this as a guide to help you find the right shade or consult your stylist. Carson's Dark & Lovely Hair Color line is made specifically for African-American hair.

300 **Q.** How do I know which shampoo and which conditioner are right for my hair type?

A. If your hair is dry, i.e. brittle, dull and has split ends, opt for a mild shampoo and a deep conditioner with lots of emollients. For damaged hair, i.e. breaks easily and is dry and breaks off when combed, choose a low pH shampoo like Professional Prescription Transpose (5.25 pH) and a deep conditioner, such as Professional Prescription Super Protein Pac, formulated for damaged hair. For excessively oily hair, common among women-of-color with a European or native American Indian background, use a shampoo with a higher concentration of detergent than conditioner, such as Revlon Herbal Deep Clean. Opt for an oil-free, leave-in conditioner for fine, thin, or delicate hair, i.e. hair that lacks body, will not hold a set and has static electricity. Select a very mild shampoo, such as Keragenics Therapy or Optimum Care Collagen Moisture and use an instant conditioner, such as Optimum Care Rich Condition or Ion Finishing Rinse.

301 Q. **How often should I shampoo and condition my hair?**

A. Every seven to 10 days is usually often enough – even if you have extensions, cornrows or dreadlocks. If you work out often or wear a wig, you may need to wash your hair more frequently. A good indication that it's time to shampoo and condition is when your hair begins to look dull, limp or when the scalp begins to itch. Use a conditioning shampoo such as Optimum Care Collagen Shampoo, Summit's Sheenique Silk Moisturizing Shampoo, Revlon's Creme of Nature or Let's Jam Shampoo. Follow with a leave-in conditioner for protection against daily abuse like sun, wind and thermal appliances. Try Fantasia IC Hair & Scalp Treatment, Sheenique Stayz-N Treatment or All Ways Natural 911 Emergency Treatment.

302 Q. **My hair is oily at the scalp but dry on the ends. What do you recommend?**

A. You're describing the natural condition of most African-American hair. The answer is to decide on a maintenance routine – shampoo, conditioner and hairdressing – based on your hair type and how you want it styled. Good products to try are Revlon's Herbal Deep Clean Shampoo or Ion Balanced Cleansing Shampoo along with Ion Moisturing Treatment or Wave Nouveau Remoisturizing Conditioner.

303 Q. What type of shampoo will rinse away heavy doses of hair lotions?

A. Use a deep-cleansing shampoo like Care Free Curl Conditioning Shampoo, Ion Balanced Cleansing Shampoo or Let's Jam Shampoo.

304 Q. What is the best type of shampoo for African-American hair?

A. Use a non-alkaline, detangling, moisturizing shampoo such as Creme of Nature, Sheenique Silk Moisturizing Shampoo or Optimum Care Collagen Moisture Shampoo.

305 Q. I am an African-American with gray hair. Is there a product that will help the yellowish tones?

A. Try one of the shampoos designed to reduce yellow or brassy tones in gray hair, such as Jheri Redding Silver Lustre or Clairol's Shimmer Lights.

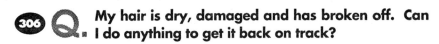

306 Q. **My hair is dry, damaged and has broken off. Can I do anything to get it back on track?**

A. It is possible to improve the look, feel and manageability of your abused tresses with conditioners and moisturizers. Try washing hair once a week, using an oil-based shampoo such as Lustrasilk Hot Oil Shampoo and moisturize with a conditioning treatment such as Sheenique Silk Reforming Complex. While the conditioner is in your hair, sit under a dryer for about 10 minutes. Set dryer on moderate to warm heat to allow hair to absorb the nutrients. Also, avoid constant use of hairsprays, or choose one that is oil-based. Brush and comb hair only when needed and be very gentle. Styling professionals sometimes recommend that their clients with damaged hair have hair extensions or style their hair in cornrows. They're a great way to give your hair a rest while keeping you well-groomed. If you do plan on wearing your hair in cornrows, make sure they are not too tight or left in too long.

307 Q. **Can black hair get bleached by the sun?**

A. Yes! Use a leave-in treatment such as Let's Jam Leave-In Treatment that has PABA as a sunscreen ingredient. Also, many finishing products like New Era Oil Sheen Spray and Fantasia's Spritz Hair Spray contain this ingredient.

308 Q. **What does castor oil do for hair?**

A. It lubricates the scalp and helps promote hair growth. Try Isoplus' Castor Oil Conditioner or All Ways Natural Castor Oil.

309 Q. If I don't want to use an oil-based moisturizer, what can I use to add moisture to my hair?

A. Try an oil-free leave-in treatment like Ion Anti Frizz Leave-In, Sheenique Stayz-N, Optimum Care Leave In or Let's Jam Leave In.

310 Q. Does black hair really benefit from those hot, concentrated conditioning treatments? If so, how would I go about giving myself one at home? Which is the right treatment for my hair type?

A. Yes, black hair can benefit greatly from hot conditioning treatments. Most professionals recommend hot conditioning treatments to their clients because heat causes the hair cuticle to open so it can absorb nutrients, vitamins, proteins and moisture that have been stripped out of the hair due to any stress. Giving yourself a deep-penetrating treatment in the comfort of your own home is easy using TCB Hot Oil or Ion Hot Oil, Let's Jam Hot Creme, Ion Effective Care Intensive Treatment or Summit's Mend Conditioner. If your hair is truly virgin, use a moisturizing treatment such as Salon Care Cholesterol Conditioner, Ion Moisturizing Treatment or Optimum Care Rich Conditioner. For best results, give yourself a hot oil treatment at home early in the evening to allow the oil to penetrate into the scalp. After shampooing your hair, apply a very warm – almost hot – conditioning treatment to scalp and hair. After 30 or 45 minutes, shampoo oil from hair and scalp, making sure all of the oil is removed.

311 Q. My hair is breaking off. What can I do?

A. Hair breaks because it is weak. Deep-penetrating protein treatments, such as Sheenique Silk Reforming Complex with Silk Amino Acids, TCB Protein conditioner, Isoplus Deep Conditioner, Proline Perm Repair, and Lekair Super Hair Repair, can begin to rebuild the strength of the hair's cortex. Use the protein treatment once a week for about a month. Then, to keep hair in good shape, use a professional leave-in conditioner such as TCB Bone Strait Nutri-Shock, Summit Penetrator 37, Infusium 23 or Sheenique Stayz-N Treatment after every shampoo.

312 Q. What is the difference between a sheen spray and a moisturizing lotion?

A. Sheen sprays only coat the hair, reflecting light to give an illusion of shine. They provide some measure of protection and make hair easier to comb. Moisturizing lotions can penetrate shaft to the hair to impart more elasticity and sheen.

313 Q. What is a wrapping lotion and when should it be used?

A. Wrapping lotions are conditioning styling lotions that are combed through the hair and molded or "wrapped" around the head to create a smooth style. Head is wrapped with a "wrap cap" and dried. Wrap is removed and hair is ready to go. Wrapping lotions can also be used for blow styling and roller setting. Try Isoplus Wrap Lotion, Lottabody Wrap'N and Tap'N or TCB Bone Strait Wrapping Lotion.

314 Q. How can I keep my hair smooth?

A. Dab pomade or styling gel just around your hairline or braids, then wrap your head with a piece of stretchy fabric or "wrap cap" for 1/2 hour.

315 Q. What kind of pomades can be used to straighten hair?

A. Pomades cannot actually straighten hair, only make it appear less curly. Often, pomades are used with a hot-comb to straighten hair.

316 Q. There are so many hairdressings. How do you know which one is right for you?

A. It all depends on why you use a hairdressing. If all you want is a healthy sheen, a sheen spray is the best choice. It moisturizes, but does not hold. Lotion from hairdressings moisturize and add some body at the same time. Grease has the consistency of Vaseline, so it can hold sculpted hairstyles. A pomade is the thickest in texture. Examples of some of the many hairdressings available, by type, include: sheen sprays – Isoplus Oil Sheen, Sheenique Oil Sheen and Revlon Finisheen; lotion or creme hairdressings – Luster's Pink Oil Moisturizer, Lustrasilk Moisture Max Lotion and Dark & Lovely Oil Moisturizer Lotion; grease – TCB Hair & Scalp Conditioner; Sheenique Scalp & Root Nourishment, African Pride Herbal Miracle Gro and Always Natural Indian Hemp Conditioner; and pomades – Sportin' Wave Gel Pomade, Murray's Hair Pomade, Dax Bergamot pomade and Pro-line Comb-Thru Gel Pomade.

317 Q. What is a good holding spray with low alcohol?

A. Hairsprays without alcohol generally do not hold as well or dry as fast; however, if you want a low alcohol hairspray, try Aura Witch Hazel Hair Spray or Resque Alcohol Free Hair Spray.

318 Q. I've worn my hair in cornrows for years, but lately I've noticed hair around my hairline is getting thinner. What is wrong?

A. It is possible that your cornrows are pulled back or braided too tightly. Keep cornrows moisturized with a spray made specifically for braids like African Pride's Braid Spray. Stress typically occurs along the hairline and breakage and thinning can occur over time. Give hair a rest from braids.

319 Q. I use a pomade for shine on my hair, but it makes my hair so stiff. What can I do to get shine without stiffiness?

A. Try a hair shiner for control and shine without stiffness, such as Jheri Redding Replenishing Hair Shiner, Aphogee Gloss Therapy or TCB Bone Strait Liquid Sheen. For a little more hold with shine, try one of the "ringing gels" like Let's Jam Shining & Conditioning Gel or Bone Strait Shining Gel. (The gel rings when the side of the jar is tapped.)

320 Q. I live in a humid climate and my braided styles tend to frizz. What can I do to help the frizziness?

A. Try a braid spray such as African Pride Braid Spray or a hair glosser like Ion Anti Frizz Glosser or Aphogee Gloss Therapy.

321 Q. Is there a specific styling aid I should put into my hair prior to braiding?

A. Try African Pride Braid Spray, Sheenique Nubian Silk Oil Treatment, Kemi Oyl, Let's Jam Conditioning and Shining Gel or Pure Shine Slicking Gel to help make braiding easier.

322 Q. What can I use to help comb through very curly hair that I don't want to relax?

A. Use a hairdressing daily that is right for you and a rinse-out conditioner after shampooing for detangling. Try Creme Of Nature Fanti or Kente Hairdress, Pro-line Comb-Thru Softener, Liv Creme Hairdress or Optimum Care Light Control Treatment. For detangling, try these rinse-out conditioners: Optimum Care Rich Condition, Ion Moisturizing Treatment, Jheri Redding Humectin Conditioner and Queen Helene Creamy Cholesterol Conditioner.

323 Q. No matter how much pomade, hairspray, gel, or mousse I put in my hair, it remains dull. What can I use to make my hair shiny?

A. Applying certain hair styling products to the hair can add luster; however, too much of a good thing can turn into a dull problem. For beautiful, shiny hair, shampoo hair with a deep-cleansing shampoo or clarifying shampoo, such as Care Free Curl Conditioning Shampoo, Ion Balanced Cleansing Shampoo or Ion Clarifying Shampoo to remove build-up. Then, moisturize with a high-protein conditioner and finish by rinsing with cool water. Use styling products sparingly. Try using high-sheen hair glossers, such as Ion Anti Frizz Glosser, Hask Pure Shine, Let's Jam Oil Free Shine, Aphogee Gloss Therapy or Bone Strait Liquid Sheen. Use just a dab!

324 Q. What gels and hairsprays won't flake?

A. Higher contents of resin will cause gels to flake. Look for a regular hold gel like Pre Con Gel Regular Hold or Isoplus Light Styling Gel. In sprays, try Summit Pre Con Spritz, Luster's Pink Oil Holding Spray or Optimum Care Soft Holding Spritz.

325 Q. Can I use styling aids not made especially for black hair? If so, which types?

A. Yes, but avoid anything with excessive alcohol or resin content. Try Ion Anti Frizz Gel Mist which doesn't contain alcohol. It's crystal clear, won't flake and contains aloe vera for extra protection.

326 Q. I recently had extensions put in my hair. How can I take care of them and my natural hair underneath?

A. To keep your hair looking beautiful, shampoo every week with a diluted pH-balanced shampoo, being careful not to massage scalp. For best results when shampooing, wet your scalp well before you lather. Rinse well, blot out excess moisture and pat your scalp with a towel. Dry braids by moving the towel downward. Next, apply a leave-in conditioner. Pat excess with a towel, leaving most of the conditioner in the hair. Then, tie on a cotton scarf and let dry completely. This will help keep braids looking neat. To prevent flaking or itching, oil the scalp with a natural oil like Sheenique Nubian Silk Oil. Between shampoos, spray on an oil-sheen. Shampoos to try include Ion Balanced Cleansing Shampoo, Care Free Curl Conditioning Shampoo and Revlon Herbal Deep Clean Shampoo. For a leave-in conditioner, try Sheenique Stayz-N Treatment, Penetrator 37 or TCB Bone Strait Nutr-Shock.

327 Q. I love the latest hairstyles with large French twists, banana rolls and upsweeps. Is there any way I can get my medium-length hair to resemble these styles without investing in a hair weave or buying a wig?

A. The fastest and easiest way to look like you have hair long enough for many of these popular styles is to purchase a hair ratt. Popular in the 1930s and 1940s, a hair ratt is a lightweight, soft plastic mesh bun that comes in several shapes, sizes and colors. To wear one, select a ratt that matches your hair color. Place it where you want your twist. Roll, or upsweep hair to cover it, and secure with bobby pins. A dab of styling gel smoothed on will help keep it looking sleek.

328 Q. Which types of combs and brushes are best for African-American hair?

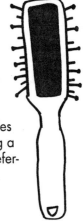

A. Select a comb made of a top grade plastic and brushes that you can pull through easily, without snagging hair. Brushes with smooth, pure boar bristles are usually the best choice instead of plastic or nylon bristles that can have rough edges. When selecting a comb, look for one with wide teeth and preferably coated as the tips (double-dipped) for extra smoothness.

329 Q. What comb or pick should I use for permed or relaxed hair?

A. Use a wide-tooth comb or pick, preferably one coated at the tips. Try the versatile "Super Styler" comb with a double-sided comb and a pick on one end. All teeth are dipped to protect from snagging hair.

330 Q. **What's the right way to straighten my hair with a hot comb?**

A. The best time to press hair is after you've washed and conditioned it. The hair must be completely dry. Place hot comb
in a heater or on a flame. Section hair into
several small portions. Apply a pressing oil,
such as Sheenique Nubian Silk Oil
Treatment or Isoplus Pressing Oil, to the
scalp and distribute through the hair evenly
and sparingly. Place the hot comb on a tis-
sue paper to test if it's too hot. If the paper
scorches, the comb is too hot to use on the
hair and should be allowed to cool. Test
until the comb leaves no brown marks on the
paper. When the comb is at the right temperature, hold section of hair upward from
scalp. Pull comb through hair quickly and
gently. Make sure hair is touched by the
back of the comb (the back rod does the
actual pressing). For best results, bring the
comb through each tress twice on top and
once on the bottom. Repeat throughout hair.
Afterwards apply a bit of hairdressing to the
scalp. Brush through. Comb and style. The Gold N' Hot
Comb has a variable temperature controlrheostat that helps
take the guess work out of the right temperature. It goes
from 145 to 320 degrees.

331 Q. Each morning, I curl my hair with an electric curling iron set on high. Does black hair require very high heat settings?

A. If you can effectively curl your hair on a lower heat setting, do so. Over time, hot curling will damage the hair. Use a protective treatment or styling product which offers some thermal protection, such as Lottabody Styling Lotion, Luster's Pink Oil Sheen Spray, Isoplus Hot, Hot, Hot Curler.

332 Q. Can I use a hot comb on chemically treated hair?

A. Yes. It is important to use a lower heat setting and always use a protective, leave-in treatment prior to use. If hair is damaged, it is not recommended.

333 Q. What type of straightening appliance should I use?

A. Try an electric straightening comb or flat iron such as those by Gold N' Hot. They're convenient and easy to use.

334 Q. What is the best curling iron size to use for black hair?

A. Size depends on the length of hair, the desired fullness or tightness of curl.

335 Q. What is the best way to dry black hair without taking out the curl or producing frizz?

A. Use a blow-dryer diffuser, with the temperature set on "cool."

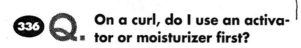

336 Q. On a curl, do I use an activator or moisturizer first?

A. For a new curl perm, apply the moisturizer first, which helps combat the drying effect a curl has on hair. Then, follow a program of applying an activator every morning to "activate" the curl pattern and using a moisturizer about twice a week.

337 Q. What can I put on my curl so it doesn't look wet?

A. Try a lighter formula activator and moisturizer like Wave Nouveau Finishing Mist and Lotion or Care Free Curl Gold Activator.

338 Q. Can people who aren't black use "ethnic products"?

A. Yes! The use of these products doesn't really have as much to do with a person's race or ethnic origin as the shape and texture of their hair. Those with very curly or very coarse hair may only be able to get the styling results they want with a black hair care product.

BEAUTY DIARY

WOMEN OF COLOR

_____

_____

_____

_____

_____

_____

_____

_____

_____

_____

_____

_____

_____

_____

_____

_____

_____

_____

_____

_____

_____

_____

Hair Color Cues

D o blonds have more fun? While the answer today would most likely be, "Not necessarily," you probably could not convince the fair-haired heroes of Ancient Greece and Rome.

Most Grecian heroes sported light-colored locks, relying on harsh soaps and bleaches from Phoenicia to lighten and redden their hair.

In the 4th Century B.C., the Athenian dramatist, Mendener, wrote that the sun's rays were the best means of lightening a man's hair. He described how hair was washed with an ointment made in Athens that turned the hair golden blond when a man would sit in the sun.

But fair hair was not the color of choice for all societies. The first-century Romans favored dark hair produced by a black dye made of boiled walnuts and leeks. Early Saxon men dyed their hair and beards blue, red, green or orange.

During the era of Elizabeth I, reddish-orange hair was in vogue for men and women. And in the days of French tyrant Marie Antoinette, pastel tresses prevailed. Hair then was heavily powdered in shades of blue, pink, violet, yellow and pure white, with each color having its own heyday.

The first safe commercial haircolor was, in fact, born in France in 1909 when French chemist

---

F.Y. 👁

Options on Color

Do you want permanent or semi-permanent color? Your stylist is the best person to help you make this selection, however, choosing one type of hair color over another depends on several factors. If you have more than 25 percent gray hair, for example, your stylist may suggest permanent haircolor to cover it. If you want your hair lightened, permanent color is generally a "must." Permanent haircolor grows out before it washes out! But, if you just want to experiment and try something different, you could try a temporary rinse that would darken blond hair, or add highlights to darker shades. A temporary rinse lasts until your next shampoo. For longer lasting color, your stylist may use a semi-permanent haircolor which lasts through at least six shampoos. If hair is fragile, or not in tip-top shape, a semi-permanent or in-between color generally will be gentler than permanent haircolor. In-between type colors are between permanent and semi-permanent. It contains no ammonia and will not lift color, so it is as gentle as semi-permanent color. Yet, it lasts almost as long as permanent color–up to 25 to 30 shampoos. The most stressful process on hair is a double process in which hair is bleached first, then colored.

Eugene Schueller created a mixture based on a new chemical, paraphenylenediamine. This concoction became the foundation of his company, the French Harmless Hair Dye Company. The name changed a year later to one of the best known names in the beauty business, L'Oreal.

What launched the modern day business of haircolor can be attributed to that American innovation, advertising. Thanks to Clairol and its campaign, "Does She or Doesn't She," coloring the hair became commonplace for millions of women, and certainly, the foundation of many salon businesses.

Prior to Clairol's ad campaign, only about seven percent of American women were coloring their hair in 1950. Today, that number has grown to more than 75 percent, and is expected to increase even more as hair coloring improves and becomes less time-consuming and healthier for hair. As more and more women – and men – go gray, haircolor could become as common as a haircut!

 Q. What guidelines should be followed in choosing a haircolor?

A. Choose a color close to your natural shade. Consider your skin tone and eye color. Haircolor with warm tones, i.e. red, gold, and auburn shades, are more compatible with warm skin tones and someone with brown, green or green-hazel eyes. These colors of eyes have the presence of yellow. Cool-tone colors, i.e. lighter gold or ash, are more suitable to fair-skinned or sallow-skin tones. Eyes are usually light to dark blue or hazel-gray, with no yellow. Make a subtle change first. You can always go more daring the next time!

340 Q. What does the term "semi-permanent" mean?

A. "Semi-permanent" means the haircolor penetrates the hair only slightly. A true semi-permanent color lasts only six to eight shampoos and will not completely cover gray, unless you use a very dark color. The clue is semi-permanent haircolor is not mixed with a developer. Long-lasting semi-permanent haircolor lasts 25 to 30 shampoos and is mixed with a developer (peroxide), but it does not contain ammonia so it cannot change your natural color. It can cover gray, but cannot make hair color lighter.

341 Q. My stylist used a double process on my hair. What is this?

A. Double process means hair was pre-lightened or bleached, then a toner was used to control unwanted red or gold tones.

342 Q. What is the difference between frosting, tipping and streaking?

A. Frosting involves pulling several fine strands of hair through a frosting cap and using bleach to remove the color. Tipping is a process in which only the tip ends of different strands of hair are bleached. Streaking or painting means to apply color or bleach with a color brush, much like painting. These processes are also known as highlighting which can also be done with squares of foil or other material.

F.Y. 👁

Terms of the Trade

When having hair colored for the first time, your stylist may use some unfamiliar terms. First, he or she will determine the **"level"** of your hair, which is the depth of your hair color shade, whether it is light, medium or dark. Levels range from 1 (black hair) to 10 (lightest blond). Then, the tone, which is the base shade of your hair at the time your hair will be colored, must be established. Tones range from warmest red to coolest ash. Tone is an indicator of how warm or cool hair color is, and it is often referred to as the hair's **"base color."** There are about a half-dozen different tones. When your hair is **"lifted,"** this means that your natural color is lightened so that the new color can be deposited into the hair shaft. When permanent color is deposited in one step, the process is a one-step or **"single process."** A **"double process"** involves first lightening the hair with bleach, which changes the level of the (continued on next page)

343 **Q.** **My hair has a tendency to feel like straw after it has been colored. What can I use to soften it?**

A. Try a post-treatment like Keragenics Rejuvenator Treatment or Aphogee Pro Vitamin Treatment. Post treatments are made to counteract brittle hair and color fading. They are basically leave-in conditioners with extra ingredients, such as silicone, citric acid, cationic sur-factants, keratin or naturally derived oils, which are designed to seal the cuticle and lower the hair's pH level to normal after a color service.

haircolor. The second process is applying new color to achieve the new desired tone. When a color product is used after bleaching, it is often called a **"toner."** Generally, the toner is a permanent color, but semipermanent and the new **"in-between"** type of color products can be used as toners, too.

344 **Q.** **How can I get a natural look when coloring my gray hair?**

A. Have your stylist help you choose haircolor a shade lighter than your natural color. This will blend better and won't result in that all-one-color look that says, "I dyed it."

345 **Q.** **What is color glossing and how long will it last?**

A. Color glossing is a shimmer of color achieved by using permanent haircolor mixed with a developer (peroxide) and conditioner. It is left on the hair a short time, usually 15 minutes. The result is a hint of color that also masks gray. It usually lasts for 10 to 15 shampoos. Again, this should be used by a salon professional as the proper shade selection is critical.

346 **Q.** I am a brunette. Can I have my hair highlighted?

A. Brunettes can have wonderful highlights. Highlighting can be achieved by applying bleach to those areas where lightness is desired. A powder bleach can be used for this service as long as it is "off the scalp" work. Another option is to frost or foil highlight with a lightener, resulting in a soft gold. Then overlay the entire head with a long-lasting semi-permanent haircolor. Overlay with a color several shades lighter than your natural color. It is best to consult your stylist for highlights.

347 **Q.** Is henna the only natural plant dye?

A. Henna is a vegetable-based dye which is made into a paste with water and then applied to the hair to create a strong, primarily red-orange shade that lasts as long as semi-permanent color. Henna coats the hair so thoroughly that it builds up over time, and it can interfere with perming or relaxing, as well as other types of color. Synthetic henna products include Ardell Hennalucent which is compatible with all chemical salon services because it does not coat the hair.

348 **Q.** What are lead acetate dyes?

A. There are few successful lead dyes in the professional market. Two common types are Youth Hair and Grecian Formula. These colors are applied frequently to the hair to "build up" or coat the hair. However, sometimes this adhering process results in "off tones," such as green!

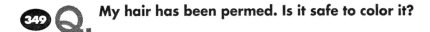

349 Q. My hair has been permed. Is it safe to color it?

A. Yes. Semi-permanent colors work very well with permed hair.

350 Q. What kind of "shelf life" do haircolor products have?

A. Haircolors used to have freshness dates stamped on them. Some still do, but manufacturer testing has shown that the shelf life of haircolor is almost unlimited if the bottle has never been opened.

351 Q. Is there a way to remove permanent haircolor?

A. This is tricky. A color remover is used when artificial color needs to be removed from the hair. It requires more "lift" than either bleaching or a permanent tint can provide. The products that remove the permanent haircolor are powerful and can only be purchased and used by a salon professional.

352 Q. What is the least harmful way to color my hair?

A. Semi-permanent haircolors do not chemically change the hair shaft and are considered to be less damaging to hair.

353 Q. What are vegetable glazes?

A. These semi-permanent glazes provide a slight change of color, designed to last two to six weeks. They give hair shine and body and are usually activated by heat; i.e, five to ten minutes under a dryer produces a temporary color reflection, 15 to 20 minutes offers semi-permanent color and 30 to 45 minutes makes color last six to eight weeks. Glazes, like Ardell's Lights and Brights, can enhance color or just provide healthy shine.

354 Q. Can I use permanent haircolor on eyelashes and brows?

A. There are special products designed specifically for coloring eyebrows and lashes. Ask your stylist to color your brows at the time you are having your hair colored. Regular permanent, semi-permanent or in-between type haircolor should not be used, however, because they can be very harmful if they get in the eyes.

355 Q. How often can I color my hair?

A. Hair can be colored as long as the hair fiber is strong and the scalp is not sensitive. If hair is spongy or breaks easily, use a semi-permanent haircolor formulated for damaged hair and begin a rigorous conditioning program. Generally, touch-ups should be done every four to five weeks, depending on the growth of the hair. If you begin to get the "zebra stripe" effect, you know you have waited too long!

356 Q. I would like to experiment with a new haircolor. What will give me a bit of color, yet not be permanent?

A. Use a temporary rinse to change the tone of your hair color and to blend gray. You could try Fancifull Mousse or Fancifull Rinse.

357 Q. What can I expect from temporary color?

A. Temporary color does not penetrate the cortex. Instead, it coats the outside of the hair shaft so it will wash out in one or two shampoos. Temporary color is great for last-minute touch-ups before a big party or to "make do" between appointments with your stylist.

358 Q. How long does a color rinse last?

A. A rinse is considered temporary haircolor, which means the color does not penetrate the hair shaft. Color rinses generally last only through one to two shampoos. Although there is no chemical reaction, if hair is damaged and porous, the color can penetrate and stain the hair. Be sure to use a color you won't regret!

359 Q. I will be attending a costume party and want to spray my hair gold. What kind of product will not damage my hair, and how can I get the spray out of my hair before going to work the next day?

A. For special events, use a spray haircolor available in an aerosol can. These products come in many colors, including gold and silver. They are temporary colors which come out completely after the first shampoo.

360 **Q.** **How long before the wedding should the bride-to-be have her hair colored?**

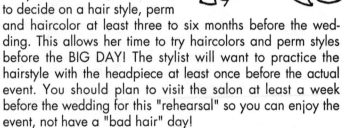

A. Brides-to-be should experiment with haircolor and a perm at least once before the wedding. Since color is performed every six weeks and hair is permed once every three months, a bride needs to decide on a hair style, perm and haircolor at least three to six months before the wedding. This allows her time to try haircolors and perm styles before the BIG DAY! The stylist will want to practice the hairstyle with the headpiece at least once before the actual event. You should plan to visit the salon at least a week before the wedding for this "rehearsal" so you can enjoy the event, not have a "bad hair" day!

361 **Q.** **In addition to a rinse, what other temporary colors are available?**

A. Colored mousses and color sprays can change a look temporarily.

362 **Q.** **My stylist lightened my hair and it turned out red! What can I do?**

A. Your stylist may choose a new haircolor and try again. To neutralize the unwanted red, he or she will use a shade with a blue or green base at the same level. You will probably require a shorter processing time, because the first color application will have increased your hair's porosity. It will be important that your stylist check every minute to ensure the desired results have been achieved. Be sure you consult a professional, as this is no time for amateur hour!

363 Q. I had my hair lightened and don't like it. Can I go back immediately to my original color?

A. Yes. The trick is, the bleaching has lifted much, if not all, of your natural color. In addition, the color service has increased the porosity of your hair. For these reasons, most color manufacturers recommend using a color filler first. The new color should be one, or even two, levels lighter than your natural hair color, because if your hair has been lighter for some time, going back to your "true color" will seem a lot darker than you may remember it. It's safer to go a little lighter than your natural color for the best overall effect.

364 Q. I am having my hair colored an auburn shade, but do not want an orange halo around my hair line. What can I do?

A. When coloring hair, many stylists will use a chemical buffer in a gel or cream form which keeps the chemicals from running and prevents stains on the skin.

365 Q. My hair has been permed and colored, but the color is fading and I have dark roots. What can my stylist do that will not dry my hair out, yet will get my color back in shape?

A. Your stylist can use a permanent haircolor on the roots only and match that same color with a semi-permanent color on the rest of the hair. Because your hair will be more porous on the ends than the new growth, the semi-permanent color will be more gentle to the hair than the permanent color.

366 **Q.** My hair was highlighted too much and I look like I have white hair. What can I do?

A. Your stylist can weave low lights through your hair which involves weaving darker strands through the hair.

367 **Q.** I would like to go blond, but do not want to bleach my hair. Is this possible?

A. That depends on your natural hair color. Black, dark brown or even medium-brown hair will require pre-bleaching. Without it, the hair would just turn orange! It is possible to go from light-brown to blonde with a "high-lift" tint that lightens up to five levels of color.

368 **Q.** I would like to be a blond for a day. What is the best way to achieve this?

A. With today's high-lift tints, just about anything is possible! But just for a day is probably not a wise undertaking. Use a spray-on color, but if you want it permanent, trust your fate to an experienced professional colorist.

369 Q. I have dark roots, even though my hair is naturally blond, and I do not want to color my hair. What can be done to blend my dark roots with the rest of my natural hair color?

A. Your stylist can apply large patches of highlighting at the roots to blend them with the rest of your hair. After adding color, each section of hair is wrapped in foil and then exposed to a heat lamp to let the color penetrate. These warm, blond, color-correcting highlights will blend the dark roots into the rest of the hair.

370 Q. My hair is dark brown and boring! I want to do something different but not drastic. What are some options?

A. Your stylist can use a double process by first using an all-over gel color to make hair look more vibrant, then applying highlights to achieve a richer, multi-toned look. The result is hair color with depth that looks sun-kissed! This is a complicated process best left to a skilled professional colorist.

371 Q. My dirty-blond hair is flat and dull-looking. How can I give it some "umph"?

A. Your hair may need luster and highlighting can achieve this. Your stylist can apply highlights to thin strands of hair around your face or may opt to do color weaving which involves applying two different shades of highlights (one slightly lighter than the other). The highlights will last until hair grows out.

372 Q. Where should highlights be applied?

A. For a subtle effect, highlights are placed on the hair around the face. For a brighter look, apply them throughout the hair.

373 Q. Recently, I ran into a long-lost friend whose red hair looked fabulous. However, she was definitely not the same strawberry blond I knew in school. What did she do to her hair?

A. She most likely had a single process haircolor, because a single process using a permanent or semi-permanent color all over the head produces vivid changes. Generally, for the most dramatic change, the stylist will color hair three shades away from the hair's natural color.

374 Q. I'm getting a two-toned effect with my haircolor after four weeks. Should haircolor last longer than this?

A. How long haircolor lasts depends on how porous the hair is, how much gray it contains, and how fast it grows. The color may fade if the hair is permed or even if you use a shampoo that is too harsh. As a rule, hair should be re-colored before there is more than one-half inch of new growth. Always use a mild, color-safe shampoo like Keragenics Shampoo Therapy or Quantum Shampoo for Permed or Color-Treated hair.

375 Q. My hair needs coloring, but is already so dry that I don't want to risk damaging it further. What can I do?

A. Precondition with a deep-penetrating moisturizing treatment or protein treatment before coloring. Then, consult your stylist for haircolor. Next, decide what you want the color to do – cover gray, lighten your natural color, lighten selected strands. Pick the appropriate type of coloring, such as semi-permanent to cover gray; permanent haircolor to lighten your own color, change its color, and add shine; or highlighting to add dimension and shine without compromising hair strength.

376 Q. Can semi-permanent color be used over permanent haircolor?

A. Generally, you cannot use most semi-permanent haircolor over permanent color. The two are designed for different porosities. However, a long-lasting semi-permanent haircolor can be used to refresh hair that has been colored with permanent haircolor because these colors are created for the same degree of porosity. Be sure to consult your stylist.

377 Q. I've heard lemon juice can be used to lighten hair. Is this true?

A. Lemon juice is not a good substitute for good haircolor. What it does is break down the hair shaft, literally resulting in a split hair shaft, not just split ends.

378 Q. I am pregnant. Can I have my hair colored?

A. Haircolor is completely safe during pregnancy. However, consult your doctor regarding the effects any medications may have on your hair color.

379 Q. My scalp itches badly when I have my hair colored. What should my stylist do to prevent this?

A. You could be especially sensitive to the haircolor. Your stylist can do a patch test 24 hours before using the haircolor to determine if it is a problem with the color product. Apply a small bit of color to the inside of the elbow. If redness, itching, swelling or irritation occurs, do not use the product. There are additives for haircolor that lessen the burning or irritation of haircolor. Your stylist can opt for a gentler product, such as a semi-permanent color.

380 Q. Can two colors be mixed together?

A. Yes, as long as they are the same type of color, i.e. semi-permanent with semi-permanent or vice versa, and of the same brand. Experimentation with haircolor should be left to the professionals.

381 Q. What type of color should be used to cover gray hair?

A. That depends on how much gray is in the hair. If hair is only five to 10 percent gray, a rinse is sufficient, or perhaps a semi-permanent color. For 10 to 25 percent gray, you'll need at least a semi-permanent color or possibly an "in between" type. If hair is more than 25 percent gray, a permanent color is required for good coverage. Cream colors in tubes with their thicker consistency often offer somewhat better gray coverage than liquids. Consider, the higher the percentage of gray, the lighter the final color. If hair is one-third or more gray, some colorists recommend mixing in some of the next deeper level of the same tone to achieve the desired results. If you want to simply blend, rather than cover gray, this can be achieved by coloring the hair a level, or even two, lighter which creates natural-looking highlights. This will also require less touching up.

382 Q. What can I do about the brassy yellow tinge to my gray hair?

A. "Brassy" is a tough term to describe. This yellowish or orange tone looks unflatteringly harsh and has many causes, including over-exposure to the sun, wind or salt water. Your stylist may use a permanent or semi-permanent color product to neutralize the yellow. This is usually one with a violet base, or possibly a blue base if the brassy tone is more orange, and at the same level as your natural color. The simplest solution may be to use a blue or violet-based highlighting shampoo to neutralize the brassiness, such as Shimmer Lights or Aura Blue Malva.

383 Q. **What do I use to get the green out of my hair?**

A. Usually, a green cast means hair was over-porous or so fine that it grabbed too much of an ash (green-based) color. You must neutralize the green with the color that is opposite it on the color wheel, i.e. red neutralizes green and vice versa. Your stylist will choose a different shade with a red or red-orange base. The new color should be at the same level as the existing color.

384 Q. **My haircolor is fading. How can I boost the color?**

A. Use a color-enhancing shampoo which is designed to freshen or tone the hair. Try Shimmer Lights Regular, Shimmer Lights Gold, or Aura Shampoos–Camomile for blonds, Clove for brunettes, Madder Root for redheads, Black Malva for black hair and Blue Malva for gray or platinum hair.

385 Q. **In the summer, my hair lightens naturally under the sun. What can I use in the winter to lighten my hair like this?**

A. Lightener products developed as gentle lighteners are recommended. Try Sun Go Lightly Maximum Strength.

386 Q. **What haircolor product will make my hair shine without damaging it?**

A. Ardell's Lights and Brights is a natural product that will add subtle highlights and lots of shine.

387 Q. I love my new haircolor. What can my stylist do that will help lengthen the time my new color lasts?

A. Many stylists will apply a clear color gloss over the hair, such as Clairol Jazzing, which not only helps to further seal the cuticle, but also extends the life of your new hair color. These glosses can be semi-permanent when used with heat or temporary without heat. They are actually very healthy for color-treated hair because they leave hair shiny, and can tone down intensity or modify color on porous hair.

388 Q. My hair grows so fast that a week after my color was put on, my gray roots started showing. What's the quick solution?

A. For spot retouching, try haircolor crayons. They are moistened and applied directly to the roots or hairline, then blended. They work like lipstick for your hair! Best bets are Tween Time Crayon by Roux.

389 Q. Whenever I have my hair colored, I end up getting the haircolor under my finger nails. What will remove this dark stain?

A. Stain removers, such as Roux's Clean Touch, will remove stains under your nails or around the hairline. You can also use a product for the nails called Gena "Nail Brite."

Q. **390** **Why does my new haircolor differ from what my stylist showed me on the haircolor chart?**

A. Most color samples are designed to give you an idea of how the color would look on white hair, since about 80 percent of people color their hair to cover gray. Gray hair is a mixture of one's original color and hair that's gone white. The reason your new hair color is different than the color swatches could be due to the fact that your own hair color, mixed with the new haircolor, created a blended shade. There could be additional reasons as well, such as condition of hair, method of application, etc. Ask you stylist.

BEAUTY DIARY

HAIR COLOR CUES

_____

_____

_____

_____

_____

_____

_____

_____

_____

_____

_____

_____

_____

_____

_____

_____

_____

_____

_____

_____

_____

Nail It

The art of well-manicured nails can be traced as far back as 4,000 years ago in southern Babylonia where the well-groomed noblemen of that time used solid gold implements to manicure their fingers and toenails.

Fingernail polish, however, is believed to have been invented by the Chinese by 3,000 B.C. as a means of indicating one's social status. A 15th century Ming Dynasty manuscript describes how the royal colors for fingernails were black and red.

Egyptians, too, indulged in the art of manicuring and coloring the fingernails, with red being the most important color of social rank. Queen Nefertiti painted her fingernails and toenails ruby red, although Cleopatra, that early beauty queen, preferred a deep russet. Even men painted their nails. It was common for military commanders of ancient Rome and Egypt to have their nails painted to match their lips before they dashed off to the latest battle.

Today, well-manicured nails are as much a part of good grooming as brushing one's teeth or combing the hair. Thanks to modern technology and continual improvements within the nail care industry, the art of manicuring can be at the finger tips of almost everyone!

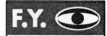

Facts About Formaldehyde

Formaldehyde is found in a surprising number of things we use everyday–even clothing! Most nail polishes and many nail strengtheners contain formaldehyde because it helps polish adhere better, and it is very effective at penetrating and hardening the nail plate. A very small percentage of people experience an allergic reaction to formaldehyde after repeated use. Over time, it can have a drying effect on anyone's nails, which is one more reason to moisturize and nourish with a cuticle conditioner regularly. The U.S. Food and Drug Administration allows the use of formaldehyde in nail care products but limits the amount permitted to only five percent. If you are concerned about possible sensitivity, there are several formaldehyde-free polishes and nail treatments available. In general, if it s not overused, formaldehyde has no harmful effects on nails.

391 Q. How do I maintain great looking hands?

A. For natural nails, the basic routine should include a cuticle oil or cream and a professional nail strengthening treatment. It's a good idea to have a medium and fine grit file. If you wear polish, you'll need a basecoat, topcoat, polish remover, polish dryer and professional formula nail polish. If you don't wear polish, use a nail buffer to maintain natural shine. You can also treat yourself to a manicure soak, a hot oil treatment, or a paraffin wrap. If you choose to extend your nail length with tips, wraps, gels or sculptured nails, use products containing botanical oils to moisturize hands and nails. Avoid products containing mineral oils, since they can cause nail extensions to lift. Basic items for nail grooming include: Contours Botanical Nail Oil, Beauty Secrets Dual Treatment Kit, Beauty Secrets Cushion White Files in medium or fine grit and Beauty Secrets Nail Enamel Dryer Spray.

392 Q. How often should I get a professional manicure?

A. This depends on your lifestyle and preference. If you prefer absolutely perfect, medium-to-long nails everyday, you'll need a professional manicure once a week. If you favor shorter length nails for an active lifestyle, you can do polish touch-ups at home. You may need a professional manicure only every two weeks. The faster your nails grow and the more abuse they withstand, the more often you'll need professional maintenance. Apply a protective topcoat every two to three days, like Beauty Secrets Dual Treatment, Orly's Top 2 Bottom or Nail Selective's Nail Radiant Top Coat Treatment to maintain your manicure.

393 Q. What products are available for home use to maintain a professional manicure?

A. There are literally hundreds of products. To help prevent breakage, try Beauty Secrets Nail Hardener and Thickener or Revlon Salon Professional Nail Revitalizer. To condition cuticles, try Contours Botanical Oil or Beauty Secrets Cuticle Oil. For base coats and top coats, try Brucci Basecoat, Nail Selectives Hydra-Coat Base Coat or Nail Selectives Radiant Top Coat. Professional nail polishes from Beauty Secrets, Nina, Brucci, Revlon and Theons often last longer than the "drugstore" variety. To remove polish, try Beauty Secrets Acetone, Non-Acetone or Adios Acetone or Non-Acetone polish removers. Dry polish with Nail Selectives Rush Polish Dry/Topcoat, Ultra Set Nail Polish Drying System, Orly Nail Spritz, Varoom or Beauty Secrets Nail Enamel Dryer Spray. Add nail buffers and nail files, and you're set to keep those nails looking nifty!

394 Q. How long should a professional manicure last?

A. Generally, from one to two weeks. A lot of this depends on how fast your nails grow and what you put them through. The faster they grow and the more abuse they withstand, the more often you'll need professional maintenance.

395 Q. Should I give my nails a "breather" between manicures?

A. The idea of leaving nails unpolished for a few days to let them rest is a common myth. Fingernails are made of dead skin cells and they don't need to breathe.

396 Q. Is it better to touch up my nail polish between manicures or completely remove all the polish to re-polish?

A. It's easier and more convenient to touch up the polish on the free edge of your nails between manicures. A manicure will always look fresher if you have the time to completely remove the polish and re-apply fresh basecoat, polish and topcoat.

397 Q. Is it essential to have nails manicured in a salon?

A. Not essential, but certainly beneficial in more ways than one! Most salon atmospheres are clean, efficient and offer a luxury we all crave – pampering! Treating yourself to a day, or even an hour, at a salon is a refreshing, revitalizing experience. With today's industry standards for salon sanitation and advances in salon technology, the salon is the best environment for nail services.

398 Q. How can I give myself a salon-perfect manicure at home?

A. A salon-perfect manicure can only be given by a trained professional. But to approximate a professional manicure or to maintain your salon manicure at home, follow these steps: The basic manicure begins by removing any old polish and cleaning the hands and nails with a nail scrub. Trim and file the nails to the approximate desired length and shape with nail scissors or clippers and medium to fine grit files. Soften the cuticles with a manicure soak and push them back with a cuticle pusher. Moisturize and nourish cuticles with a cuticle cream or oil. If you wear polish, you'll use one coat of basecoat, two coats of polish and one coat of topcoat polish dryer. If you don't wear polish, use a nail buffer to smooth small ridges and maintain natural shine.

399 Q. I have scraggly cuticles. How can I get them back in shape?

A. Massage cuticle cream, oil or lotion into the cuticle. Then,use a cuticle stick to gently push back the cuticle after you have softened it, which in most cases eliminates the need to trim the cuticle. If necessary, cuticle trimming should be left to the professional, who will use special stainless steel cuticle trimmers which come in different "jaw" sizes. Best bets are Tweezerman "Pushy" Cuticle Pusher, Winning Nails Plastic Cuticle Pusher, Flowery Thin Manicure Sticks and Tweezerman Cuticle Scissors.

400 Q. What is the best way to remove hangnails?

A. Nail technicians remove hangnails with cuticle nippers. The best way to prevent hangnails is to use cuticle creme, oil or lotion that is massaged into the cuticle and nail mantle. Then use a cuticle stick to gently push back the cuticle after you have softened it, which in most cases eliminates the need to trim cuticles of hangnails.

401 Q. I was a chronic nail biter, but have stopped. My habit has made my cuticles uneven. Is there anything I can do to even out my cuticles?

A. Have regular manicures, including cuticle cream, oil or lotion that is massaged into the cuticle and mantle. Then use a cuticle stick to gently push back the cuticle. To condition the cuticles, try European Secrets Intensive Cuticle Care Treatment II.

402 Q. What causes puffy cuticles?

A. Puffy cuticles can be caused by several things. If the cuticle has been scraped, or there are abrasions on the cuticle and chemicals are then used, this could irritate the skin. Puffy cuticles can also be caused by an allergic reaction to products used on the nails or to products in which the hands are being soaked. Your professional nail technician can best diagnose the reason for your puffy cuticles and assist with treatment. Professional application of nail products is the best prevention for skin irritation.

403 Q. My cuticles seem to peel after a professional manicure. What can I use to prevent this?

A. When cuticles peel between manicures, this generally indicates extra dry skin. Proper home maintenance can ensure longer wearability of a professional manicure. By regularly massaging cuticle oils and conditioners into the base of the cuticle area, you can help prevent problems like cuticle peeling. Best bets are Contours Botanical Oil or Perfect Nail's Caviar Bead.

404 Q. What can I use to keep my cuticles from growing so fast?

A. If necessary, cuticle trimming should be left to the professional who will use special stainless steel cuticle trimmers which come in different "jaw" sizes. However, you can massage Varoom Lemon Brite Cuticle Remover, Winning Nails Cuticle Creme, Adios Creamy Cuticle Remover or Claire Topper Cuticle Remover into the cuticle and mantle, then use a cuticle stick to gently push back the cuticle.

405 **Q.** What is the most important product that I should buy to keep my cuticles in shape?

A. There are two types of cuticle oils and conditioners that can be used. Cuticle conditioners that contain mineral oil, like Winning Nails Cuticle Cream, should only be used on natural nails to soften the cuticles and prevent hangnails. Cuticle conditioners that contain botanical oils can be used on all nails, including nail extensions, to soften cuticles and prevent hangnails. Try Contours Botanical Nail Oil, Perfect Nail Caviar Beads, Revlon Salon Professional Cuticle Perfector or Beauty Secrets Nail Matrix Fortifier. Cuticle conditioners that contain mineral oil should never be used with nail extensions because they may cause lifting.

406 **Q.** There are so many types of nail files. How do I know which one to use for which purpose?

A. Choose your file depending on how you plan to use it. The higher the grit number, the smoother the file. Coarse files (80-120 grit) are best for use on acrylic extensions. Medium files (150-180 grit) are best to shape extensions of medium thickness, like most tips and wraps and to shape the free edge of natural nails. Fine files (200-240 grit) are best for removing small bumps, ridges or discoloration and shaping the free edge on the natural nail.

407 **Q.** My nails are very thick and difficult to shape. Is there anything I can use to thin them?

A. The best solution for shaping thick nails is to use a medium grit file on the free edge. Frequently, thick nails also have ridges. Natural nail buffers (fine grit) can be used to reduce ridges on the nail surface for the appearance of a thinner, smoother natural nail.

Q. **What is a circular nail disk?**

A. The circular nail disk, commonly referred to as the Round Buffer or Disk File, is used in different ways, determined by the grits of the file. A higher number grit (or a softer buffer) may be used on the surface of the natural nail and nail extensions. The curve of the round disk buffer helps to prevent scraping the cuticle and allows for a natural filing motion on the surface of the nail. A lower number grit (or a coarser file) may be used on the surface of nail extensions with extra care. Both round buffers can be folded in half to file the underside of a tip for better adhesion. Tropical Shine makes circular nail disks in blue (medium grit), pink (fine grit) and black (combo grits).

Q. **How do I use a small, four-sided nail board?**

A. The four-section nail buffing board can be used on both nail extensions and natural nails. Begin with the most coarse section, which is usually black. Finish with the smoothest section, which is usually grey. This buffer removes imperfections in the nail and buffs to a smooth, glossy shine. Try Tropical Shine 4-in-1 Buffer.

Q. **Is it better to use a metal file or an emery board? Why?**

A. Metal files or emery boards can be used to shape the free edge of the fingernail by filing corner-to-center in one direction, never filing from side-to-side on a natural nail, which may weaken the stress points of the free edge. A metal file or emery board should not be used on the surface of a natural nail because these files are usually too coarse. There are many kinds of non-metal files available, as metal tends to cause nail splitting.

411 **Q.** How do I use a nail buffer, and is it healthy for my nails?

A. A nail buffer can be used on both nail extensions and natural nails without harm. Begin with the most coarse section which is usually black. Finish with the smoothest section, which is usually gray. This buffer removes imperfections on the natural nail and nail extensions, and results in a smooth, glossy shine. Best bets are Tropical Shine 3-way and 4-way. A natural chamois skin buffer is used with a buffing creme like Winning Nails. For buffers, try Perfect Nails Chamois Stik or Winning Nails Chamois Buffer.

412 **Q.** Is there any special type of nail file that can be used on nails that are soft?

A. A fine-grit nail file (240 grit) is excellent for shaping the free edge of soft nails. It is also the first step in removing scratches, ridges or imperfections from the natural nail surface by using a three or four-sided buffer.

413 **Q.** What is the best nail length for someone with short fingers?

A. Nail length is not necessarily determined by the shape or length of the fingers. People with short fingers normally have shorter nail beds, so a medium-to-short length for natural nails is best. If nail extensions are preferred, a shorter-to-medium length extension is best because nails that are too long on a short nail bed will not be well-balanced with the length of the nail bed and free edge.

414 Q. I have big, athletic hands. What is the best nail length for me?

A. People with larger hands normally have medium-to-larger nail beds, so a medium length for natural nails is best unless a very active life style requires a shorter length. If nail extensions are preferred, depending on the life style, a shorter-to-medium length extension is best. Depending on a person's life style, most nail extensions work well as long as you keep a shorter-to-medium length. Nail tips now come in a variety of lengths and styles to suit all life styles and preferences.

415 Q. What is the best length for a bride-to-be?

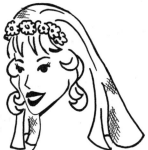

A. That depends on personal preference and life style. On this very special day, you tend to be hard on your nails. With little or no time for maintenance, a shorter or medium length nail is preferable.

416 Q. I have nail ridges. What causes this problem and can it be fixed?

A. There are many different causes of nail ridges. Trauma to the nail, certain medications taken over long periods of time, and chronic health conditions can cause temporary or permanent nail ridges. If ridges are temporary, they will grow out within six months to a year. Use nail strengtheners and ridge fillers as well as cuticle softeners to promote healthy new growth. If the ridges are permanent, continuous use of a natural nail buffer or chamois skin buffer and buffing cream like Winning Nails, as well as a ridge filler, will smooth the appearance of ridges. Try Beauty Secrets Ridge Filler, Brucci Ridge Filler or Nail Selectives Silkfill Ridgefiller.

417 Q. I have always buffed the top of my nails to smooth unwanted ridges. Is there a product that will fill in the ridges and leave a smooth finish?

A. Yes! These products are called ridge fillers and are designed to fill in the ridges and imperfections on the natural nail. They should be used on a regular basis because most ridges are imperfections of the natural nail. Natural nail buffers can be used in conjunction with ridge fillers for the perfect finish to a smooth nail. Try Orly Ridge Filler Primer Base Coat or Super Nail Fiber Nail Wrap.

418 Q. I have rough nails with ridges. What can I do to camouflage these imperfections when I wear pale pink polish?

A. Use a ridge filler as a basecoat to fill in ridges and smooth out the surface of rough nails before applying polish. Also, use a natural nail buffer in conjunction with a ridge filler to leave the appearance of a smooth natural nail. Try Brucci Ridge Filler, Orly Ridgefiller Primer Basecoat or Nail Selectives Silkfill Ridgefiller.

419 Q. Can I use a topcoat as a basecoat or vice versa?

A. Probably not. Although they look similar, these two products are designed to do different things. Basecoats are usually thicker and stickier, which helps the nail polish adhere better, and they contain more resins to give the nail added strength. Topcoats on the other hand, are thinner and contain more ingredients that create a durable surface on the nail, they are made to add strength, dry quickly and protect the polish from daily wear and tear. There are a few time-saving combination basecoat/topcoats on the market, but usually the two are not formulated to be interchangeable. Try Nail Selectives Hydra-Coat Base Coat or Nail Selectives Radiant Top Coat. For a combination basecoat/topcoat, try Orly Top 2 Bottom or Beauty Secrets Base/Topcoat/Clear.

420 Q. Recently, all my nail polish peeled off in one large piece after a professional manicure. What caused this, and how can I prevent this from occurring?

A. It is very unusual for polish to peel in one large piece. If it does occur, these may be some of the reasons: an oil or creme was applied to the nail and not rinsed off, the base coat and polish were not compatible or a quick-dry polish (looks like basecoat) was used instead of a base coat.

421 Q. What is a nail strengthener?

A. Strengthening treatments are also called nail hardeners, and they are formulated to strengthen the nail plate. The nail plate is made of keratin, the same protein as hair. Some strengtheners actually penetrate into the nail plate to strengthen nails from the inside. These strengtheners often contain formaldehyde to penetrate and harden nails. Protein strengtheners work in a similar way and contain a protein such as collagen. Other hardeners, like a liquid wrap, work on the surface of the nail plate. They contain tiny fibers of a fabric, like nylon, to coat nails for extra thickness. Nail vitamins can always be used in addition to your manicure routine. Nail strengthening treatments to try include Beauty Secrets Nail Hardener and Thickener, Contours "Ten Natural Nails," Brucci Miracle Formaldehyde-Free Nail Hardener, SuperNail Fiber Nail Wrap (liquid wrap) and Windsor Nail Nutrition Tablets (vitamins).

422 Q. I've had the flu, and my nails are weak and brittle. What can I do to make them "well"?

A. Weak nails usually need more nourishment or more strength. By using a nail strengthening treatment, nails build up as they grow out. Cuticle conditioners will nourish the nail, since healthy nail growth begins beneath the cuticle. Good skin care can help too. Professional skin moistruizing lotions and creams should be a part of every basic manicure routine. Nurse your nails back to health with Beauty Secrets Dual Treatment Kit, Delore Onymyrrh, Revlon Salon Professional NailBuilder, Nail Nutrition Tablets or Nail Selectives Rebuild Fortifier.

423 Q. How do I get my nails to grow faster?

A. There is no "sure thing" to make nails grow faster. The average adult's nails grow one-eighth of an inch per month. The right diet and proper maintenance are your best bet for healthy nails. Nail vitamins, cuticle conditioners and nail strengtheners all can help promote healthy new growth. Consider using Windsor Nail Vitamins, Revlon Salon Professional Cuticle Gel, Revlon Salon Professional Nail Builder (which contains calcium), Nail Selectives Rebuild Fortifier or Formula 10 Nail Strengthener.

424 Q. Do nail growth products work?

A. Products applied to the surface of the nail plate do not affect nail growth, because nail growth begins at the matrix of the nail (commonly referred to as the "mother of the nail") deep inside the finger. Massaging cuticle oil or cream into the base of the nail every day will help to stimulate circulation in the nail growth area to promote nail growth. Good products to try include: Beauty Secrets Nail Matrix Fortifier, Nail Selectives Rebuild Fortifier, Beauty Secrets Dual Treatment Kit or Contours Botanical Oil.

425 Q. My nails will grow to a certain length but then begin to chip near the tips. What can I use to strengthen them?

A. Nails that chip are caused by a number of different things, but usually they need more nourishment or more strength. By using a nail strengthening treatment, nails build up as they grow out. A cuticle conditioner will nourish the nail, since healthy growth begins beneath the cuticle. Good skin care can help too. Professional skin moisturizing lotions and creams should be part of every basic manicure routine. Natural nail buffers will smooth the chips and peeling on the free edge of the nail to preserve the length until the nail grows out. Nail vitamins can always be used in addition to your manicure routine.Strengthening products include Delore Onymyrrh, Brucci Miracle Nail Hardener Formaldehyde Free, Windsor Nail Nutrition Tablets and Nail Selectives Rebuild Fortifier.

426 Q. How can I prevent my nail polish from chipping two or three days after my professional manicure?

A. Proper home maintenance can ensure longer wearability of a professional manicure. Use products such as cuticle oils or conditioners, professional polishes, topcoats and nail buffers. To prevent chipping, try Brucci Acrylic Shield, Delore Chip Proof, Wet Look Glaze and Revlon Professional Energized Topcoat.

427 **Q.** **What is the best nail color for small hands?**

A. All well-manicured natural nails or nail extensions, on small or large hands, can wear any shade that best complements your skin tone. If you have blue tones in your skin, choose shades with a blue base, like rose or plum shades. If you have yellow tones in your skin, select shades with a yellow/orange base such as corals, oranges, tomato-reds. Do not wear red nail polish on nails that are bitten. If you are uncomfortable with color, sheer shades look very natural.

428 **Q.** **What is the best nail color for long fingers?**

A. All well-manicured natural nails or nail extensions, on small or large hands, can wear any shade that best complements your skin tone.

429 **Q.** **I love bright red polish, but not long nails. Can I wear red on short nails?**

A. Certainly! Pick a shade that complements your skin tone, and for best results, use a professional polish such as Beauty Secrets Polish, Nina Polish, Revlon Polish, Brucci Polish or Theons.

430 Q. What is the difference between a French Manicure and an American Manicure?

A. In contrast to the stark white tips and "painted" look of French Manicures, the American Manicure Natural Look Polish System gives both nail extensions and natural nails the authentic look of perfectly healthy bare nails wearing only a clear topcoat. Both Orly and Nina make products for a French Manicure.

431 Q. When polishing my nails, what is the best way to achieve an opaque look with the pale polish?

A. To achieve an opaque look, follow this procedure: First, apply a coat of basecoat; then apply a coat or two of white polish. Apply a single coat of desired color, then finish with topcoat.

432 Q. Which is more drying to my nails, frosted or matte polish?

A. Because the basic ingredients in frosted and matte polish are the same, neither is more drying to the nails.

433 Q. What is Toluene?

A. Toluene is an organic solvent that is used in nail polishes, top-coats and basecoats to help the polish stay on the nail. Toluene is included in a list of hazardous chemicals cited in a 1987 California law. A study conducted by the CTFA (Cosmetics, Toiletry and Fragrance Association) produced evidence that the amount of toluene found in nail polish is 10 times below the maximum amount allowed by California law. In other words, the amount of toluene in nail polish does not pose a threat to users. If you are looking for toluene-free nail products try Revlon's new Salon Professional Nail Enamel or Nail Selectives 3/4 oz. Nail Treatments.

434 Q. How many coats of polish are best for a perfect manicure?

A. For best performance, we recommend one basecoat, two coats of your choice of polish and one topcoat.

435 Q. My polish bubbles up? What causes this?

A. Several factors can cause nail polish "bubbles." First, be sure to use a professional quality polish. Second, check the age of your polish – old polish will thicken and cause bubbling. Polish thinners are available, but a new bottle is best. Third, never shake your polish bottle because the beads in the bottle can create bubbles. Instead, roll the bottle between your hands. Fourth, if you use a spray-on nail polish dryer, don't hold it too close to the nail or over-spray. Finally, be sure the first coat of polish is completely dry before applying another coat. To thin polish, try Adios Polish Thinner.

436 Q. How long does it take to completely dry polish?

A. How long it takes depends on the type of polish and polish dryer. Generally, it takes one to two hours before nail polish is completely dry. Formaldehyde-free polishes take more time to dry. Many nail polish dryers allow you to use your hands five to 15 minutes after polish is applied. However, that doesn't mean heavy gardening!

437 Q.: How long should nails dry after a manicure before typing or using a computer?

A.: Today, many nail polish dryers are available that allow you to begin typing or using your computer five to 15 minutes after your polish is applied. There are topcoat polish-drying systems brushed on over the polish color to protect polish and speed up drying time, as well as light-drying systems, many of which require the use of a specific topcoat and/or basecoat. Do not mix and match different systems, and be sure to follow manufacturer's instructions. Nail drying machines dry polish gently and efficiently with the use of cool or warm air. There are also spray and brush-on polish dryers of the oil-base type, used on top of the final coat of polish to set it, or the oil-free variety, used between coats of polish to speed drying time.

438 Q.: The only time I have to polish my nails is at night before bed. How do I prevent "sheet marks" without losing my sleep?

A.: Today, many nail polish dryers are available that will allow you to sleep soundly five to 15 minutes after your polish is applied. Best bests for sleeping soundly are Varoom Speed Dry, Nail Selective's Rush Super Quick Pro-Dry/Topcoat, Contours Polish Dry and Beauty Secrets Fast Finish 60 Second Polish Dryer/Topcoat.

439 Q.: How long must I wait before taking a bath after I've had a manicure?

A.: To prevent smudging, it is best to wait one to two hours before hopping in the tub or shower. A topcoat polish dryer, such as Nail Selectives Rush Super Quick Pro-Dry or Varoom Speed Dry will help nail polish dry faster.

440 Q. How can I get rid of smudges without doing a complete manicure?

A. Try Claire Topper's Nail Triage which will smooth out little smudges and chips to make your manicure last longer.

441 Q. I want to do something really unusual with my nails. What's a good option to try for special occasions?

A. Try Nail Art! Beyond polish, there are a myriad of products for decorating nails. This is called "nail art," some of which, like airbrushing, take a great deal of skill and are left to the professional. There are a variety of products that make nail art easy for almost anyone. Decals are probably the easiest way to create multi-colored designs that look almost like airbrushing. Some come with adhesive backing; others need to be moistened with water. They must be applied to clean, dry nails which may be previously polished. Foil nail decorations are applied by first coating the nail with a specially formulated glue, sometimes called a foil emulsion. Then, the dull side of the foil is pressed onto the nail. When it's lifted away, the colorful side shows. One or more colors of foil can be used together for a "mosaic" effect. Most nail art decoration must be sealed with a special topcoat, often called a bonder or sealer. Follow the manufacturer's instructions exactly for best results. If you want to try nail art yourself, check out Winning Nails 4-Color Airbrush Lace and Foil Decals, Cina Nail Jewelry Decals, Cina Foil Mosaic Kit, Cina Rhinestones, Cina Try Me Nail Art Kit, Eimsuk Fine Art Nail Decals, and Cina Top Coat and Bonder or Winning Nails Tough Coat Bonder/Sealer.

442 Q. Can I use a regular topcoat instead of a bonder for applying nail art?

A. It depends on the topcoat. If it is an especially thick formula, it will probably be sufficient to protect the jewelry or decals and keep them in place. It is always best to use the specific bonder or sealer made by the nail art manufacturer.

443 Q. Are decorative nails proper for a wedding, and what types are available?

A. There are a variety of products that make nail art easy for almost anyone. From decals to foil nail decorations. Also available are festive lace, pearl and gemstone designs, which are designed with the sophistication appropriate for a day as important as your wedding. A recommended style for your wedding day is soft and subtle. Remember to follow manufacturer's instructions. For wedding-appropriate designs, try Winning Nails Lace Decals, Foil Decals, and Eimsuk Fine Art Nail Decals for Wedding.

444 Q. What are the pros and cons of having acrylic nails?

A. Acrylic nails, in most cases, are the strongest semi-permanent nail extensions available. As with all nail extensions, with proper application and proper maintenance there are virtually no negatives to wearing acrylics.

445 Q. My nails won't grow past my fingertips without breaking off. Are fake nails right for me?

A. Today, nail extensions can accommodate all life styles. Nail extensions are not thick and do not have to be worn long. Today, a more natural look is appealing and extensions are versatile enough to express your personal style. Beautiful, well-maintained nails are the finishing touch to a complete look. There are many different types of extensions available such as tips, sculptured nails, nail wraps and gel nails. Consult a professional nail technician to determine which nail extension is best for you.

446 Q. Should my manicurist mix and match liquids and powders from different manufacturers to create my sculptured acrylic nails?

A. NO! Each acrylic system has it's own chemical formulation, and the individual components are balanced to work together. If a powder from one manufacturer is used with liquid from another, the nails may take too long to set up; or they may set up too fast and become brittle. Sometimes, combining products that aren't meant to work together can cause uncomfortable heat sensations.

447 Q. I just had my acrylic nails (tips or wraps) removed and my nails feel as thin as eggshells. What will strengthen them?

A. If the extensions were removed properly, the eggshell feeling will be temporary. Use a nail strengthener to help toughen them up. Nail and cuticle oils will help plump the layers of the natural nail that have been repeatedly dehydrated by the use of antiseptics in the process of applying extensions. To strengthen nails, try Nail Selectives Rebuild Fortifier or Beauty Secrets Dual Nail Treatment Development System. Contours Botanical Oil helps rehydrate nails. If the nails were removed improperly, the nails won't just feel thin – they'll be thin! Every time a nail extension is picked off, pulled off or bitten off, two to three layers of the natural nail plate are forcibly removed. This can actually remove half the thickness of the natural nail! To ensure proper removal of extensions, see your nail professional.

448 Q. I wear extensions, but they keep lifting up. What's wrong?

A. There are many possible reasons, such as nails shaped with deep indentations or unusually high arches; not using an antiseptic to clean, sanitize and dehydrate the natural nail before applying the nail extension; using products with mineral oil and lanolin on hands; not pushing back the cuticle properly when applying extensions; or taking certain prescription medications. Hormonal changes in the body (such as menopause), as well as excessive stress can also contribute to lifting. When applying nail tips, be sure to select the correct size and use a good nail glue. If the glue looks stringy it is too old and won't work properly. On acrylic nails, be sure to use non-acetone polish removers because acetone may cause them to lift. Apply the acrylic properly. Acrylic nails are best applied by a professional manicurist.

449 **Q.** What's the difference between a linen, silk or fiberglass wrap? Is one better or stronger than the other?

A. Linen provides excellent strength but is not very thin or transparent. Silk looks the most natural and offers the flexibility, but may be too delicate for people who are hard on their hands. Fiberglass provides the best of both worlds with the natural look of silk, plus the strength of linen. Silk and fiberglass often come with an adhesive backing, available in sheets, strips and pre-cut fingers. Try Beauty Secrets Silk or Fiberglass Nail Wrap Kits or Gena Brush On Fiberglass Wrap System.

450 **Q.** What is the difference between a liquid nail wrap and a silk or linen nail wrap?

A. A liquid wrap contains tiny fibers of a fabric, like nylon, so it's a little like a "nail wrap in a bottle." It coats nails to give them extra thickness to reinforce them. Liquid wraps are great for easy maintenance and quick repairs on natural nails. A fabric nail wrap is a semi-permanent nail extension. A thin layer of fabric is cut to size and glued onto the nail to add strength, and sometimes length. Wraps can be done on natural nails or as a tip overlay, which is the most common application. Usually, one layer of fabric is applied and then one or more layers of glue are applied on top of it. Try Super Nail Liquid Wrap, Orly's Romeo Instant Nail Wrap or Nutress Liquid Silk Wrap.

451 **Q.** **What is nail wrapping?**

A. A nail wrap is a semi-permanent nail extension that is a thin layer of silk, linen or fiberglass or fabric, cut to size and glued onto the nail to add strength, and sometimes length. Wraps can be done on natural nails or, as a tip overlay, which is the most common application. Usually, one layer of fabric is applied and then one or more layers of glue are applied on top to provide strength.

452 **Q.** **My nails are constantly splitting. Is there a product that can protect my nails?**

A. Nail care products containing nylon fibers which, when applied to the natural nail, can provide external thickening and temporary strengthening. Since the added strength is temporary, it is recommended these products be applied with every manicure to provide consistent strength as your nails grow longer. Try SuperNail Fiber Nail Wrap with Fibers or Nail Selectives Silk Fill.

453 **Q.** **I'm worried about getting infection from a manicure. What should my manicurist do to prevent the spread of infection?**

A. The best insurance against infection is for your manicurist to previously sanitize each implement that will be used during your manicure, also to cleanse and dehydrate your natural nails as extra security. If you think you have a fungal infection, tell your manicurist. She should not apply nail extension products.

454 Q. **Can I use regular nail glue to fill in my gel extensions?**

A. Nail glues and no-light gels are chemically similar in that they are both cyanoacrylates, but they have different viscosities. Therefore, it won't do any damage to interchange them, but to ensure the best results, it is always best to repair and fill gel extensions with the same gel used to create them. To fill gel extensions, try Gena Brush-On Nail Gel System, Gena Brush-On No-Light Nail Gel or Super Nail No-Lite Gel. Gel extensions applied using an ultra violet light contain a different chemical, so you should not use regular nail glue on them.

455 Q. **One of my nails looked green after I removed the acrylic over the nail.**

A. Water molds are bacterial infections. They turn the nail plate green or brownish. This particular condition is caused by moisture being trapped between an extension and the natural nail plate due to nail extensions lifting because of improper application and maintenance. There are products available, such as Beauty Secrets Nail Antiseptic and OrigiNails Steri-Nail, which cause the water mold to be dormant. During this time, with special care taken by your nail technician, the green discoloration will grow off.

456 Q.: How can I tell if I have nail fungus? Should I discontinue my manicures?

A.: Nail fungus is a severe bacterial infection which is often contagious. Nail fungus makes the nail bed white and flaky. This condition can be caused by injury to the nail or improper application or maintenance of nail extensions. To prevent nail fungus, properly dehydrate the natural nail with a nail antiseptic before any extension products are applied. The second step in preventing nail fungus is proper application. If products are applied improperly, the nail extensions will lift and leave the nail susceptible to fungal infection. There are antifungal nail treatments and products on the market, such as No Lift Nails "Fung Off", OrigiNails "Steri-Nail", Pro-Tect Antifungal Nail Oil and Beauty Secrets Nail Antiseptic. If you think you have a fungal infection, consult with your nail technician and physician, since fungal infections can be serious and highly contagious.

457 Q.: What is the best antiseptic for use on your manicure tools?

A.: There are several implement sanitizing products on the market, such as Wahl Clini-Clip Clipper Blade Disinfectant, Oster Spray Disinfectant and Barbacide. Be certain to read the package and follow the manufacturer's instructions carefully.

458 Q.: What is the difference between acetone and non-acetone nail polish remover? Which is best?

A.: Acetone polish removers are for use on natural nails. Non-acetone polish removers contain ethyl acetate or nethyl ethyl keytone as their active ingredient and were developed for use with nail extensions because acetone can cause extensions to become brittle and "lift."

459 Q. **What is the best type of nail polish remover to use? Do those that claim to be conditioners really have any benefit?**

A. Acetone polish removers are for use on natural nails. Non-acetone polish removers contain ethyl acetate or nethyl ethyl keytone as their active ingredient and were developed for use with nail extensions because acetone can cause extensions to become brittle and "lift". Conditioning agents are added to polish removers to counteract the drying effects of the solvents which come in contact with your skin and nails when removing polish. Try Gena Zip Off Nail Polish Remover.

460 Q. **How can a pedicure keep my feet healthy?**

A. Regular pedicures will keep feet looking pretty and help to prevent dry skin and eliminate callouses. Start with a 10-minute soak using a foot bath or soak. Dry skin sloughing lotions, as well as special foot files will remove dry skin and callouses. Pedicure lotions, powders and cooling gels (a refreshing treatment) are all available for pampering purposes. In addition, there are special antiseptic, antifungal foot sprays available if treatment for fungus is necessary. A coarse grit file can be useful for tough toenails. And a professional quality polish is the finishing touch for any good pedicure. Perfect Feet offers a complete line of professional pedicure products.

461 Q. I have callouses and thickened skin on my heels. How can I get rid of this unsightly problem?

A. Treat yourself to a regular pedicure. Use a sloughing lotion or special foot file to remove dry skin and callouses. Using these regularly will begin to eliminate those callouses. Also, using a pumice stone can greatly reduce unsightly callouses and dry patches. Try Gena's "Perfect Feet Pedicure" System, Winning Nails Fancy Foot Pedicure File and Tweezerman Pedicure Callus Shaver for extra thick skin and callouses, which safely shaves away dry, dead skin. Follow manufacturer's directions carefully.

462 Q. How should my toenails be trimmed? Straight or rounded?

A. Toenails should be trimmed and filed straight and never too short. This will help to prevent ingrown toenails.

463 Q. What is the best tool for clipping my toenails?

A. Professional heavy-duty stainless steel toenail clippers by Revlon or Tweezerman should be used because of the thickness of the toenail.

464 Q. Can fingernails and toenails get sunburned?

A. No, natural nails and toenails do not get sunburned. Polished nails that are not coated with a topcoat that contains a UV inhibitor can turn yellow and discolor the polish. UV-inhibiting topcoats include Beauty Secrets Fast Finish and Beauty Secrets Nail Hardener and Thickener.

465 Q. My toe nails turn yellow. What should I do to whiten them?

A. Yellow and stained toe nails can be caused by wearing polish without a basecoat, or your nails may appear yellow if you've worn clear or sheer polishes without a UV inhibitor in the sun. A consultation with your nail professional can help determine the cause. Use Gena's Nail Brite Whitening Scrub which contains a mild abrasive or Varoom Lemon Brite Cuticle Remover which contains an ingredient like lemon juice to easily eliminate discoloration.

466 Q. How can I prevent my pale nail polish from turning yellow in the sun?

A. Polish topcoats that contain an ultra violet inhibitor to prevent lighter polishes from changing colors or turning yellow include Beauty Secrets Nail Hardener and Thickener, Beauty Secrets Fast Finish Dryer/Topcoat and Nail Selectives Crystal Nail Builder.

467 Q. When I remove my red nail polish, my nails seem to stay pink for weeks. Is there a product available that will take the stain off?

A. The pink discoloration on the natural nail is due to the pigmentation of the red polish. To help prevent discoloration, use a professional basecoat. To remove the stain from the natural nail use Gena's Nail Brite. Stain-preventing basecoats include Nail Selectives Hydra-Coat Base Coat, Orly Top 2 Bottom, Brucci Base Coat and Revlon Salon Professional Stain Guard Base Coat.

468 **Q.** I am a lifeguard and am consequently in the sun a lot. What can I do to keep my nails from yellowing?

A. There are polish topcoats available that contain an ultra violet inhibitor to help prevent natural nails from yellowing. Also, these topcoats help prevent lighter polishes from changing colors or turning yellow. Try Beauty Secrets Fast Finish or Beauty Secrets Nail Hardener and Thickener.

469 **Q.** I have stopped and started smoking numerous times in the past 20 years. Each time I start and stop smoking again, I notice that my nails yellow. Is this possible, and what can I do to correct it?

A. Yellow and stained nails can be caused by smoking or by wearing polish without a basecoat. Your nails may appear yellow if you've worn clear or sheer polishes without a UV inhibitor in the sun. A consultation with your nail professional can help determine the cause. A thorough buffing with a fine grit nail file may be enough to remove the yellow. If not, use a nail scrub which contains a mild abrasive or use Gena's Nail Brite Whitening Scrub which contains an ingredient, like lemon juice, to easily eliminate discoloration.

470 **Q.** **What's the quickest and best way to fix a broken nail?**

A. There are many quick-mending products available for natural nails, such as nail glues. If the natural nail is split, there are products that can mend the natural nail that are applied to the surface and are temporary. If the natural nail is broken there are products that can be used to extend the length of the nail as a temporary fix. If you are wearing nail extensions and one breaks, "emergency repair" kits are available for quick fixes, but it is always best to have your professional nail technician repair and maintain your nails. For emergencies, keep on hand Beauty Secrets Antifungal Nail Glue, Beauty Secrets Wrap Kits in Silk or Fiberglass, 5-Second Nail Repair Kit or the Nails-To-Go Travel Repair Kit.

471 **Q.** **What is a pumice stone?**

A. Pumice is a light, porous stone, formed by the escape of steam from cooling volcanic lava. Pumice stones can be used to remove rough, dry, built-up patches or callouses, after the skin has been soaked in warm water to pre-soften. Try Flowery Pumice Stone or Burmax Italian Pumice Stone.

472 **Q.** **My manicurist warms a lotion before I soak my hands in it. Can I do the same at home to moisturize my hands and nails?**

A. Paraffin is a waxy substance used in heat treatments by manicurists and aestheticians. Warm paraffin is used to coat the hands, feet or face. This paraffin coating holds heat in for 10 to 15 minutes and causes the pores to open to allow moisturizers to penetrate into the skin more readily. Paraffin therapy conditions and softens the cuticles and leaves hands feeling soft and pampered.

473 Q. Does a moisturizer help keep nails healthy?

A. Moisture loss is a major cause of nail brittleness and breakage. A daily moistruizing treatment for hands and nails will keep moisture loss to a minimum. The more your hands and nails are exposed to drying elements (like dish washing, the sun or handling paperwork), the more frequently you should moisturize. There are cuticle oils and creams designed specifically to moisturize the cuticle. Using these products regularly also stimulates blood circulation in the matrix(where nail growth originates deep inside the finger) which helps to promote healthy nail growth. Try these moistruizing products: Contours Botanical Oils, Perfect Nail Caviar Beads or Revlon Salon Professional Cuticle and Nail Conditioner.

474 Q. What is paraffin wrap?

A. Parrafin is a waxy substance used in heat treatments by manicurists and aestheticians. Warm paraffin is used to coat the hands, feet or face. This parrafin coating holds heat in for 10 to 15 minutes and causes the pores to open to allow moisturizers to penetrate into the skin more readily. Paraffin therapy conditions and softens the cuticles and leaves hands feeling soft and pampered.

475 Q. I use hand lotion but my hands continue to get very rough and red.

A. Hands tend to get more rough and red in the winter because your hands are drier than at any other time of the year. The massaging action stimulates blood circulation throughout the hands and arms and promotes the absorption of conditioners into the skin. Be certain to apply hand creams frequently, more than once a day if your hands are very dry. Always apply creams after washing your hands or submersing them in water. Try Triple Lanolin's Hand and Nail Conditioner, MRX Hydrating Lotion or Purist Swedish Herbal Hand Cream.

BEAUTY DIARY

NAIL IT

Skin Care and Hair Removal

Ever since the days of the cave man, some form of sharp implement has been used to remove hair. From primitive sharpened flints to collections of prized bronze razors, hair removal tools have been regarded as essential to good grooming. Modern technology has made the often painful task of hair removal easier, and in many cases, much less painful, thanks to the invention of the safety razor in 1762. For centuries, women endured nicks, scrapes, and burns when having their unwanted body hair plucked, waxed, pulled and scraped off. And although in the early 20th Century women could borrow from the boys those Schick, Gillette or Sunbeam razors, it wasn't until 1940 that Remington rolled out the first electric shaver specifically designed for women. Today, in most modern societies, smooth, shiny skin is not only a sign of good health, but also good grooming. Women tweeze their eyebrows to suit the latest fashion trend. They shave, wax, and depilate hair on legs, under arms, above the lip and in the delicate "bikini" area. All in the name of "beauty."

476 Q. **What method do dermatologists recommend for removing unwanted hair?**

A. Electrolysis is suggested for sparse, unwanted hair. For more abundant hair, waxing is best. Seek a recommendation for a good electrologist from your dermatologist.

477 Q. **What is the best way to remove hair using a hand-held machine?**

A. Hair should be 1/6 to 1/2 inch long. Take a hot shower or hot bath to soften hairs. Pull skin taut while depilling hair. Consider waxing hair first, then using the machine for keeping the area hair-free as hair grows in.

478 Q. What is the difference between the paraffin used to soften hands and the wax used for hair removal?

A. Paraffin wax is lanolin-enriched and contains moisturizing oils. Gigi Honee Wax is made with clover honey and other natural resins which facilitate hair removal.

479 Q. Why does it hurt when I get my legs waxed? Can the pain be lessened?

A. Leg hair is pulled off with the wax. To help ease the pain, skin should be pulled very taut in the opposite direction from which the wax strip will be removed. Stretching the skin properly is the most important tip for reducing the pain. Immediately after the wax is removed, apply firm pressure to the area with your hands. The sting can also be lessened at the point by placing an ice-cold pack where hair was removed.

480 Q. How long should my hair be to be waxed?

A. Hair should be 1/2 inch long the first time for the wax to take hold.

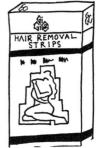

481 Q. What hair removal technique lasts the longest?

A. Waxing, especially when a warm wax is used because it penetrates into the pores and pulls out the entire hair from the root. On the average, it takes three to six weeks for the hair to grow back. For permanent hair removal, electrolysis is recommended.

482 Q. Can I wax my legs at home effectively?

A. You can wax your legs at home, but probably not as effectively as a professional can. Hot wax kits for home tend to be messy. However, Gigi Microwave Kit is an efficient system providing a transparent wax so that you can see exactly which hairs have been covered by the wax. Care should be taken in heating the wax, and be sure to follow closely the manufacturer's instructions. The Clean & Easy Mini Waxer is easy to use because the wax is applied with a roll-on applicator that eliminates mess. Hair is removed with cloth strips almost as effectively as in a professional waxing salon. You might also want to try the cold wax kits in which wax is spread on strips that you press on and tear off. The downside: sometimes not all the hair is stripped off.

483 Q. How do I get rid of ingrown hairs on my legs after I have had my legs waxed?

A. Waxing could have caused this because hair is removed below the skin line. A hair is ingrown when it re-enters the skin after it came out. To remove it, sterilize a fine sewing needle in boiling water and gently pick the hair out. If it doesn't pop out easily, give up. You may need to see a dermatologist if the hair does not grow out. To avoid the problem, don't shave too close, wax or use a depilatory.

484 Q. How long will my skin stay smooth after using a depilatory?

A. That depends on your hair type – whether you have strong, coarse or fine hair. Usually two to six weeks because depilatories reach hair just below the surface.

485 Q. Why do depilatory creams smell so badly?

A. They contain two powerful chemical compounds, sodium thioglycolate and calcium thioglycolate which both can dissolve keratin – what hair is made of. Sometimes the smell is worse after the depilatory is applied because the thioglycolate acid reacts with the hair to create a sulphur-type by-product – the bad egg smell! A few formulations are available which are not as strong smelling, such as Clean & Easy Cream Depilatory.

486 Q. What do I do if my skin breaks out after using a depilatory?

A. Wash with betadine and follow with Neosporin cream or a cortisone spray to reduce inflammation. Betadine is an anti-bacterial cleanser that is available over-the-counter from your pharmacist.

487 Q. Will depilatories dry my skin?

A. No, not if you follow up with a finishing cream or balm, such as Palm Beach Skin Saver with aloe vera to soothe and moisturize skin.

488 Q. When should I shave, morning or the night before?

A. Shave at night to reduce redness.

489 Q. When should I shave my legs before going to the beach?

A. Wait 12 hours after shaving or waxing to plunge into the spa, pool, lake or ocean. Shaving stubble is the one drawback of shaving, although it is still the most popular method for removing leg and bikini hair.

490 Q. What is the proper way to shave my legs?

A. Shave hair in the opposite direction hair grows. Use razors made for women because their curved handles are easier to hold and seem to help prevent nicks.

491 Q. How can I prevent the redness and stinging that occurs after I shave my legs?

A. Wash your razor and legs with betadine before shaving. Shave in the shower using Clubman Shave Cream which will soften the hairs and make shaving easier. After shaving, use Gigi Antiseptic Lotion to moisturize the skin. Palm Beach Skin Saver will help minimize redness and irritation and will leave skin feeling smooth and cool because it is enriched with aloe vera.

492 Q. Can I easily remove hair from the "bikini" area?

A. Shaving may be the easiest, but is not the most effective way to remove bikini area hair. The best way is to have hair professionally removed using a waxing product with azulene. If this is not possible, try Clean & Easy Bikini Roll On or Clean & Easy Wax Strips which can be used at home.

493 Q. What is the best way to remove facial hair myself?

A. Ardell Surgi-Cream dissolves the hair at the skin level. An easy-to-use solution is Gigi Removal Strips for the face.

494 Q. What is the best method to remove or minimize those unsightly hairs that grow in the nose and ears?

A. Nose hair should be clipped with tiny manicure scissors or Tweezerman's blunt nose scissors made especially for this task. For easier hair removal, Wahl makes a battery-operated nose hair trimmer. Nose hairs should not be waxed! Ear hairs can be waxed or tweezed, but it is quite uncomfortable. Most good stylists usually will clip the ear hairs when they are trimming the hair. At home, have your spouse, roommate or significant other tweeze the hairs for you, since it is hard to do it yourself.

495 Q. How do I choose tweezers? There are so many shapes?

A. For a long lasting, durable tweezer, choose a professional quality 100 percent stainless steel tweezer that will not rust when cleaned. The prongs should have a light, gentle spring action and the gripping platforms (at the tips) should be smooth and polished. When the tips are pressed together, they should meet perfectly. Tweezerman makes a variety. The most popular is Tweezerman's Slant Tweezer. Selecting the shape is a matter of personal preference.

496 Q. **What is the best way to tweeze my brows?**

A. First, brush the hairs in the direction of the hair growth. Isolate the hair you want to tweeze. Always tweeze in the direction of the hair growth. Pull ONE hair at a time, gently and smoothly. Do not yank the hair out. Ouch! Brows should start just above the inner corner of the eye and extend slightly past the outer corner of the eye. Be careful not to remove too much hair because brows that have been tweezed too much won't always grow back!

497 Q. **How can I reduce the irritation from having my brows tweezed?**

A. Dampen a cotton ball with a mild astringent, like Sea Breeze, and gently wipe the area to be tweezed to help prevent infection. Take a steamy shower or place a hot washcloth over your brow before tweezing to open the pores. Don't use an ice cube or "freeze before you tweeze," because this will close the pores and it makes it harder to pull the hair. Use a moisturizer after, not before tweezing, so you are sure to get a good grip on the hair.

498 Q. **What is the best softener for the hands?**

A. For long term moisturizing, try a salon paraffin manicure that softens skin and cuticles with moisturizing oils. For daily use, try a moisturizing lotion like Skin Saver Aloe Vera Lotion, Vienna Triple Lanolin Hand and Body Lotion or Vienna Aloe Vera Hand and Body Lotion for extra protection.

499 **Q.** Is there a difference between the natural sponges used by spas and the synthetic sponges I find at the drugstore?

A. Natural sponges are more durable than synthetic fibers, which is why you may find them at spas. They will hold up better over time.

500 **Q.** What is the difference between using a loofah and using a body cleansing grain?

A. Both exfoliate, i.e. slough off dead skin cell layers. A loofah is made from a loofa plant and is made into a cloth or mitt. Body cleansing grains contain granules which when rubbed on skin exfoliate it, allowing the body to be polished instead of just washed.

SKIN CARE AND HAIR REMOVAL

_____

_____

_____

_____

_____

_____

_____

_____

_____

_____

_____

_____

_____

_____

_____

_____

_____

_____

_____

_____

_____

_____

S K I N   C A R E   A N D   H A I R   R E M O V A L

_____

_____

_____

_____

_____

_____

_____

_____

_____

_____

_____

_____

_____

_____

_____

_____

_____

_____

_____

_____

_____

_____

_____

References

1. *"Panati's Extraordinary Origins of Everyday Things"* by Charles Panati, 1987, Harper & Row, Publishers.

2. *"Why Did They Name It?"* by Hannah Campbell, 1964, Fleet Press.

3. *"Great American Brands and Topsellers"* by David Powers Cleary, 1981, Fairchild.

4. *"The Strange Story of False Hair"* by John Woodforde, 1972, Drake.

5. *"Accessories of Dress"* by Katherine M. Lester and Bess V. Oerke, 1940, Manual Arts Press.

6. *"400 Years Without A Comb"* by Willie L. Morrow, 1984, Morrow's Marketing, Publishing, Research Development Corporation.

7. *"Living Legends in Cosmetology"* The Beginning by Carole Parks, Shoptalk, Jan./Feb. 1993.

Glossary

Acetone:
The main ingredient in nail polish removers for natural nails.

Acid Perm:
A permanent wave product with a pH around 6.5 to 8.0. Generally, acid waves are milder products, producing soft, loose, natural-looking curls.

Acrylic:
The material out of which sculptured nails are created. Acrylic is made by combining a liquid and a powder which, when brushed onto nails and allowed to dry and harden, forms a tough, artificial surface.

Activator:
In haircolor, an ingredient added to bleach which increases the speed of bleaching action without harming the hair. Activators are known by several names, including Bleach Boosters or Accelerators. In nail care, an activator speeds or controls the hardening process.

Alkaline Perm:
A permanent wave product with a pH around 7.5 to 9.5. Generally, alkaline waves are stronger products, producing firm, crisp, springy curls.

Amino Acids:
Hair and nails are made of protein, and protein is made up of these chemical "building blocks."

Ammonia:
A strong, alkaline substance found in some (but not all) permanent haircolor. Ammonia sends a chemical signal to the developer, to lighten (decolorize) the hair.

Ammonium Thioglycolate:
The active chemical ingredient in alkaline permanent waves and ethnic curl products. Nicknamed "thio" in the beauty industry.

Ash:
The term used by many manufacturers for a "cool," green-based haircolor.

Basecoat:
A clear, thick polish applied before nail color to provide a smooth surface and help the other coats of polish adhere better.

Base Cream:
A protective cream that is applied to the forehead, ears and neck before relaxing (or perming) to minimize skin contact with chemicals.

Bleach(ing):
To chemically strip some color from the hair. Also referred to as Decolorizing or Pre-lightening.

Body:
The quality of liveliness or springiness of hair.

Body Wave:
Another term for a permanent wave.

Bonding:
A temporary way to add more hair to a person's head. Locks of synthetic or human hair are attached with glue.

Botanical:
Containing plant extracts or ingredients made from plants.

Brassy:
The term for unflattering yellow, red or orange tones in some hair colors. Hair can turn "brassy" from overexposure to sun, wind or chemicals, or from lightening the hair.

Buffer (related to skin):
A thick, protective cream which can be applied to the face and skin during a color process to prevent stains.

Buffer (related to nails):
An extremely fine-grit file used for shining the surface of the nail.

Cetyl Alcohol:
An ingredient, a fatty amino acid, of some conditioners and styling aids, which smoothes and softens hair.

Chelating:
A deep-cleansing process, also known as Clarifying, to lightly strip the hair before a chemical service.

Citric Acid:
A common ingredient in post-perm treatment products, which gives hair a fresh scent and helps eliminate perm odor.

Clarifying Shampoo:
A type of shampoo designed for deep-cleansing, to remove something from the hair: chlorine, hard-water minerals or a build-up of styling aids.

Cold Wave:
Another term for an alkaline perm or curl product.

Color Filler:
A substance which can be applied during the coloring process to ensure more uniform, natural-looking results. A filler takes the place of missing color pigment in the hair.

Color Remover:
Used to remove artificial color from hair. Some color removers will take permanent color out of hair; others will only remove semi-permanent color.

Condition(ing):
To provide moisture and nutrients to the hair. Conditioning products combat dryness and make hair easier to style.

Cool:
Refers to blue, violet or green-based tones in haircolors.

Cornrows:
Fine, tight braids.

Cortex:
The middle layer of an individual hair, which makes up about three-quarters of the hairshaft. The pigment which gives hair its color is located in this layer.

Crimping Iron:
A thermal styling appliance that presses a loose, wavy pattern into hair.

Curl(ing):
A permanent wave for African-American hair.

Curl Activator (Moisturizer):
A maintenance product for chemically curled hair, to moisturize it, make the hair feel softer, and "revive" the curl.

Cuticle (related to hair):
The outer layer of the hairshaft. It is made up of multiple layers of translucent cells which overlap each other like shingles on a roof. When the layers are smooth and flat against each other, the hair reflects more light and looks shiny.

Cuticle (related to nails):
The rim of skin that surrounds the nail and prevents dirt and bacteria from getting down under it and causing infection.

Cuticle Oil (creme):
A treatment that is massaged into the cuticle area for nourishment and moisture.

Cuticle Stick:
Used to push back excess cuticle from the nail plate.

Dandruff:
Tiny flakes of dead skin cells from the scalp. There are two kinds: oily and dry dandruff. The dry kind can be caused by a build-up of hair products, like styling aids. Some types of persistent dandruff are caused by medical conditions and should be treated by doctors.

Deep-penetrating Treatment:
A conditioning product for occasional use which is more intensive than an everyday conditioner. Treatments are formulated to revive dry, brittle hair by adding protein, vitamins and moisture. Some require heat; others do not.

Disulfide Bonds:
The strongest of hair's chemical bonds, which give each hairshaft its shape. Relaxing breaks these bonds; curling disconnects and then re-shapes them.

Double Process:
A color service which requires two steps to complete: first, lightening the existing haircolor with bleach; and second, applying new color.

Elasticity:
The hair's ability to stretch without breaking and then return to its original shape. Elasticity determines how well the hair will "hold" a curl, a major factor in choosing the correct type of perm.

Enamel:
Another term for nail polish.

End Wraps (Papers):
Small squares of paper (or other fabric) used to keep the ends of a strand of hair smooth and separated as it is rolled onto a perm rod. They're used so the hair will curl evenly along its entire length.

Exothermic Perm:
A permanent wave product that creates its own heat chemically is "exothermic."

Extension:
An artificial addition which gives length to a natural nail. Nail tips and sculptured acrylic nails are all different types of extensions.

Fill (fill-in):
The regular service done to maintain artificial nails. Includes filing and/or adding more material at the back of the nail to blend in new growth.

Finishing Spray:
A hairspray with medium hold which contains enough memory resins to keep a style in place for a full day.

Flat Iron:
A thermal styling appliance that straightens hair by pressing it between two flat metal plates.

Foam Foundation:
A lightweight piece of soft foam which can be cut, shaped and pinned beneath the hair to create a bun or "roll." Also called a "ratt."

Follicle:
The passageway in the scalp through which a single shaft of hair grows out.

Formaldehyde:
A chemical used in nail polishes to make them adhere better; and strengthening treatments to penetrate and harden the nail plate.

Formaldehyde-free:
Products which do not contain formaldehyde.

Freezing Spray:
The firmest-hold type of hairspray, good for spot styling or hard-to-hold hair.

French manicure:
A style of nail polish application which uses two shades of polish, matched to the customer's skin tone, to make the nails look "natural" but flawless.

Fungus:
An infection which can grow under artificial – or even natural – nails. Nail fungus often turns the nail bed white and flaky.

Grease:
A common term for hairdressings with the consistency of Vaseline.

Grit:
The texture (coarse, medium or fine) of a nail file.

Hairdressing:
A maintenance product that adds oil to hair and the scalp, and gives the hair sheen. A hairdressing can also provide styling support, depending on its consistency.

Hairshiner:
A liquid or spray applied to styled hair to mask split ends and make the hair appear instantly shinier. Most hairshiners contain silicone which lightly coats the cuticle and "fills in" the split, damaged areas.

Hardener:
Another name for a nail strengthener.

Henna:
A vegetable dye from the henna plant which has been used since ancient times to color hair. Its dried leaves and stems are crushed into fine powder, then applied as a paste to dry hair. Traditional henna gives a reddish-orange hue.

Highlighting:
Lightening and coloring hair selectively. The technique can be done with squares of foil or other material; or a special kind of plastic "tipping cap." Small strands of hair are highlighted selectively, to create a "layered" or "sun-streaked" effect. Also known as "frosting," or "tipping."

Hydrogen Peroxide:
The chemical ingredient in a developer which, when mixed with permanent haircolor, triggers the lifting power of the tint and creation of molecules of new color. Also, the active chemical ingredient in most perm neutralizers.

Hypoallergenic:
Formulated to be less likely to cause an allergic reaction in sensitive people.

In-between Type Color:
A newer type of color product, which combines the gentleness of semi-permanent color with the long-lasting qualities of permanent color. In-between type color requires a mild catalyst to work.

Iron(ing):
A term for thermal straightening.

Keratin:
Both hair and nails are made up of this strong protein. Keratin contains 20 different amino acids.

Lacquer:
Another term for nail polish.

Level:
The depth of a haircolor's shade – whether it is light, medium or dark.

Level System:
The chart used by haircolor manufacturers to identify and label haircolor along two "dimensions." There are 10 levels (depths) of haircolor, from Level 1 (black hair) to Level 10 (lightest blonde). There are also a half-dozen or so tones, from "warmest" red to "coolest" ash.

Lift:
A comb with widely-spaced teeth used to gently pick up, raise or fluff sections of hair.

Lift (related to haircolor):
To lighten the haircolor. "High-lift" means to lighten it a lot.

Lift(ing):
Separation of an artifical nail from the natural nail, or the natural nail from the nail plate.

Liquid wrap:
A type of strengthener that contains tiny fibers of a fabric to reinforce the surface of the nail.

Lye:
The common term for a relaxer product that contains sodium hydroxide as its active chemical ingredient.

Mantle:
The skin at the base of the fingernail. The mantle is directly over the matrix.

Matrix:
The spot, just under the skin of the mantle, where the nail plate starts growing.

Melanin:
The pigment that makes up hair's natural color.

Metallic Dyes:
Comb-through hair dyes which derive their color from lead or other metallic "salts." They appear to change the hair color gradually, since they build up on the hairshaft with successive applications.

Moisturize:
To add moisture or to close the cuticle to prevent loss of moisture.

Mousse:
A styling foam which provides light hold, adding lift and fullness to hairstyles.

Nail Bed:
The skin beneath the nail plate.

Nail Plate:
The hard part of the natural nail that's usually called the "fingernail."

Nail Scrub:
A lightly abrasive nail cleanser used to remove yellowing and stains.

Nail Treatment:
One of a number of types of products designed to strengthen, nourish or protect the nails. Treatments do more than simply make nails look better; they "treat" a problem, like cracking or peeling.

Neck Strip:
A sanitary strip of paper or fabric which is wrapped around a client's neck under the towel or cape during a perm or any other chemical service.

Neutralizer:
A product applied to the hair after a chemical service, designed to stop the chemical action by counteracting alkalinity (most chemical services require an alkaline pH).

Nippers:
Tools for trimming cuticles or nails that are more precise than scissors.

No-Base Relaxer:
A relaxer which does not require application of a base cream to the entire scalp before use.

No-Lye:
The common term for a relaxer product that contains calcium hydroxide as its active chemical ingredient.

Non-acetone:
Nail polish remover that contains ethyl acetate or methyl ethyl ketone as its active ingredient instead of acetone. Recommended for use on nail extensions.

Oil Sheen:
Another term for a Sheen Spray.

PABA:
Para-Aminobenzoic Acid is a substance which absorbs ultraviolet light – it's a "sun block." PABA is used in skin and hair care products, as well as in tanning lotions.

Panthenol:
Vitamin B-5 which conditions and "plumps" the hairshaft to make it appear thicker.

Perm:
A wave or curl that is set chemically in the hair and remains generally for several months.

Perm Rejuvenator (also called a Revitalizer):

A product to help revive the curl in permed hair that is growing out. It can also help reduce frizziness in a new perm.

Perm Solution:

Another term for Waving Lotion.

Permanent Color:

Color that will grow out before it washes out because it chemically changes the natural pigment of the hair.

pH:

The degree of acidity or alkalinity of any water-based solution. A pH of 7 is neutral, on a scale from 0 (very acidic) to 14 (very alkaline). Human hair seems to thrive best at 4.5 to 6.5 – a slightly acid pH level. Permanent haircoloring is an alkaline chemical process which temporarily raises the hair's pH to 10 or 11.

Pick:

A comb with widely-spaced teeth. A pick is used more for "fluffing" a hairstyle than for actually combing or smoothing it.

Pomade:

A type of hairdressing with the thickest consistency.

Porosity:

The hair's ability to absorb moisture. Hair must be slightly porous to allow conditioners and chemicals to ease their way into the hairshaft.

Porosity Equalizer:

A product used as "insurance" prior to a color or perm service to make sure the color will come out uniformly even when some parts of the hair are more porous than others.

Post-treatment:

A conditioner or normalizing lotion used immediately after a haircolor service to close the cuticle and help "seal in" the new color.

Press(ing):

A term for thermal straightening.

Pressing Comb:

A thermal styling appliance which is pulled slowly through hair to straighten it.

Pressing Oil (Cream):
A waxy product that protects hair while it's being heat-styled and that helps hold the hair's new shape.

Pre-treatment:
A product applied to hair before a perm or color service to make it more receptive to the new perm or color.

Pre-Wrap:
A term for products applied to hair immediately before the waving lotion. Some are porosity equalizers; some pre-soften resistant hair; and others are moisturizers to protect against dryness.

Processing Cap:
A lightweight, disposable plastic cap that holds in enough natural body heat for most perm products to work.

Processing Method:
How the waving lotion works on hair during the perming process is called "processing." Most perm products process at room temperature; some require heat from a dryer.

Processing Time:
The amount of time a chemical service remains on the hair before being rinsed out.

Protein:
The substance from which hair is made. To strengthen damaged hair, some hair care products contain protein.

Re-arranger:
The first step in a curl service. This application of "thio" loosens the hair's natural curl in preparation for the waving lotion.

Relax(ing):
To permanently straighten hair with chemicals.

Resins:
The ingredients in hairsprays and styling aids which give them holding power. There are two kinds of resins in beauty products: "holding" resins, to hold hair in place; and "memory" resins, to enable the hair to return to its desired style, even after it is combed out or tousled.

Resistant:
A term for hair that is difficult to color, perm or relax, usually because it is not porous enough. The scales of the hair's cuticle lay too flat and tight against the hairshaft to allow chemicals to enter. Resistant hair must sometimes be pre-treated to get the cuticle to "open up" a bit.

Ridgefiller:
A type of basecoat which contains very fine grains of a material like talc. This material fills in ridges and small indentations in the natural nail to create a smoother surface for polishing.

Root Perm:
A perm service that is done on only the new growth of previously-permed hair that has partially grown out.

"S" Pattern:
The well-defined "S" shape that a stylist looks for when checking a test curl.

Sculptured Nails:
Extensions made from acrylic or gels.

Sebum:
The natural oil that lubricates and protects the hair and scalp.

Semi-permanent:
Haircolor that gently penetrates the cortex without lifting the natural color, and that washes out gradually. No developer is needed, making this a non-oxidative type of color.

Shape:
The term which refers to whether an individual hairshaft – or a full head of hair – is straight, wavy or very curly.

Sheen Spray:
The very lightest type of hairdressing.

Single Process:
Haircoloring that requires only one step to achieve the desired result.

Spiral Curls:
Long, corkscrew-shaped curls.

Spot Perm:
A permanent wave given on selected sections of hair instead of the entire head.

Spritz:
A spray-on styling aid. This term also describes the method of application – a light mist from a pump bottle. A spritz is different from a hairspray because it only holds a style – it doesn't "remember" it.

Stearyl Alcohol:
An ingredient of some conditioners and styling aids which smooths and softens hair.

Styling Gel:
A thick styling aid (sometimes called a "glaze") which is used for sculpting individual curls or "wet look" hairstyles.

Sunscreen:
A substance which absorbs the sun's ultraviolet (UV) light rays to prevent yellowing of the nails.

Temporary Color:
A category of color products which wash out in one or two shampoos. They include rinses, mousses, haircolor crayons and sprays.

Test Curl:
A strand of hair that is partially unwound from its perm rod to see how completely a perm has processed.

Texture:
The diameter (thickness) of the hairshaft which determines how the hair "feels" (wiry, thin, etc.) There are three basic hair textures: coarse, medium and fine.

Texturizer:
A styling aid which coats the hairshaft causing it to stiffen and increase in diameter.

Thermal Lotion:
A liquid styling aid formulated to protect hair from heat damage by hot rollers, blow dryers, curling irons, etc.

Thickener:
Also called a "texturizer."

Thio:
The term commonly used by stylists for ammonium thioglycolate (ATG), the key chemical ingredient in an alkaline perm. It's not a good expression because there are other, different types of "thio" chemicals (for example glyceryl monothioglycolate, the key ingredient in acid perms).

Tint:
A permanent color which contains ammonia, so that it lightens the existing color and deposits new color, in a single step.

Tip Overlay:
When a wrap or acrylic is applied over a nail tip to add strength and make it wear longer, the service is called a tip overlay.

Tips:
Pre-molded artificial fingernails, usually made of plastic, which are glued to natural nails.

Tone:
The indicator of how "warm" or "cool" a haircolor is. Also referred to as the hair's "base color."

Topcoat:
A clear polish applied on top of color to add shine and protect the other coats of polish from chipping.

True-to-Rod-Size:
Means that a perm product creates curls that are the same size as the rods used.

Ultraviolet (UV) light:
Can refer to light from the sun or to lamps used in salons. UV light is used to dry and harden some nail gels.

Virgin Hair:
Hair that has not been previously permed, colored, straightened or otherwise chemically treated.

Viscosity:
The thickness of a liquid; its ability to flow. The higher the viscosity, the thicker the liquid.

Volumizing:
To make hair appear thicker.

Warm:
Refers to gold, orange or red-based tones in haircolors.

Water Mold:
An infection which can grow under artificial – or even natural – nails. Watermold often turns the nail plate brown or green-ish.

Waving Lotion:
The first chemical step in the perming process. The waving lotion penetrates into hair to disconnect the chemical bonds so the hair can be reshaped.

Weave:
A temporary way to add more hair to a person's head. Strands of human or synthetic hair are sewn into place.

Weft:
A lock of synthetic or human hair used in bonding or weaving.

Working Spray:
A hairspray with the gentlest hold, typically used while hair is still being styled.

Wrap:
A small piece of fabric (silk, linen or fiberglass) which is cut to size and glued to a natural nail or nail tip to add strength and/or length.

Wrap Cap:
A head covering, usually made of nylon or silk, worn to maintain the shape of a wrapped hairstyle. Also called a "doo rag."

Wrapping:
Rolling hair onto perm rods.

Wrapping Lotion:
Setting lotion used to create a tightly-molded, wrapped hairstyle.

About The Editor

Beth Barrick-Hickey is national beauty advisor and a product development consultant to Sally Beauty Supply, the world's largest distributor of professional hair and nail care products. A 10-year veteran in the beauty business, Ms. Barrick-Hickey is founder and president of Total Marketing Productions, a consulting and trade show production company. She also is co-owner of a leading professional nail products company in Arlington, Texas.

A licensed cosmetologist and former nail technician, Ms Barrick-Hickey is well known in professional beauty circles for her education and training programs for professional nail technicians, beauty schools and professional beauty products distributors nationally and in Puerto Rico and Canada. Her dynamic personality and entertaining style have made her a popular speaker at beauty industry trade shows around the country.

The author of "New Business, How To Get It, How To Keep It" for salon professionals, Ms. Barrick-Hickey served on the board of the Nail Manufacturers Council, and is a member of the American Beauty Association (ABA), the Beauty and Barber Supply Institute (BBSI), and the National Cosmetology Association (NCA).

Prior to her professional beauty career, Ms. Barrick-Hickey was on-air talent for a cable television company where she helped develop and co-hosted a special beauty and fitness program.

A
acid: 8
Albright, Dr. Jim: 4
alcohol: 24
alkaline: 8

B
banana clip: 70
banana rolls: 132
Belson Products: 4
blotting: 19
blow dryer: 75-80
blow dryer diffuser: 136
blow dryer hoods: 82
blow dryer, hand held: 74
blow dryer, holding of: 77
blow dryer, nozzle attachments: 80
blow dryers, proper use: 76
bobby pins: 69
body cleansing grain: 191
botanical products: 13
braided styles, frizzing: 130
braiding, styling aid: 130
brassy hair: 14
Breck, John: 8, 10
bridal headpiece: 69
brush cleaner: 57
brush rollers: see rollers
brushes: 57-61
brushes, African-Americans: 133
brushes, anti-static: 58
brushes, boar bristle: 58
brushes, children's hair: 61
brushes, curly hair: 59
brushes, fine, thin hair: 60
brushes, flexible bristles: 52
brushes, gray hair: 61
brushes, hot air styling: 74, 76, 85
brushes, long hair: 60
brushes, sharing: 62
brushes, short, cropped hair: 61
brushes, straight hair: 60
brushes, "The Tong": 59

brushes, wire: 62
Bulkley, Deanna: 4

C
castor oil: 125
cetyl alcohol: 24
chignons: 69
cleansers: 8
clips, for pin curls: 69
cold wave: 96
Collier, Jeanie: 5
color glossing: 141
color rinse: 145
color-correcting highlights: 149
color: see hair color
coloring hair: see hair color
combs, African-Americans: 133
combs, for curly hair: 130
combs, for relaxed hair: 133
combs, for wet hair: 63
combs, hot for chemically treated
   hair: 135
combs, hot, for straightening hair:
   134
combs, wet: 28
combs, when to use: 62
combs, wide-tooth: 52
combs. for teasing: 63
concentrator nozzle: 82
conditioners, after coloring: 33
conditioners, after moisturizing
   shampoo: 28
conditioners, cholesterol: 22
conditioners, deep-penetrating: 22-
   23, 25
conditioners, everyday: 23, 25
conditioners, for damaged hair: 24
conditioners, for fine hair: 26
conditioners, for oily hair: 27
conditioners, for oily scalp: 24
conditioners, greasy feeling: 25
conditioners, hot oil: 22
conditioners, how often: 123

conditioners, instant: 27
conditioners, leave-in: 23, 26-28, 32
conditioners, moisturizing: 22
conditioners, no-heat activated: 34
conditioners, protein: 22-23
conditioners, rinse-out: 23, 26
conditioners, same brand as shampoo: 25
conditioners, selecting: 122
conditioners, the lowdown: 22
conditioning treatments, African-Americans: 126
cornrows, thinning hair: 129
cortex: 23
cream rinse: 23
crimping iron: 74, 76, 88
crown volume: 43
curlers, hot, for traveling: 76
curling hair: 65
curling irons: 35, 74, 84-85
curling irons, after perm: 85
curling irons, cleaning: 86
curling irons, coatings: 83
curling irons, for a wave: 84
curling irons, for black hair: 135
curling irons, for curly hair: 84
curling irons, for quick set: 86
curling irons, for tight curl: 83
curling irons, gray hair: 86
curling irons, settings for black hair: 135
curling irons, size of: 86
curling, without chemicals: 121
curls, pin: 69
curls, straightening: 111
curls, that don't look wet: 136
curls, using activator and moisturizer: 136
curly hair, straightening: 87-88
cuticles: 27
cuticles, growing too fast: 163
cuticles, peeling after manicure: 163

cuticles, products to keep in shape: 164
cuticles, puffy: 163
cuticles, scraggly: 162
cuticles, uneven: 162
cyanoacrylates: 183
cystine bonds: 94

D
dandruff: 17, 53
deep-penetrating treatment: 31-33
depilatory: 195
depilatory creams, odor: 195
depilatory, causes dry skin: 195
depilatory, causes skin to break out: 195
diffusers: 81-82
Dodson, Elaine: 4
double process: 140
dry ends: 25
dryers: see hair dryers and blow dryers
dull hair: 46
dull hair, African-Americans: 131
dyes, lead acetate: 142

E
eczema: 17
Elaine Dodson's Natural Way of Beauty Salon: 4
electric shock protectors: 92
electrolysis: 192
emollients: 9
end papers: 71
epoxy ball-tips: 57
eye brows, using tweezers: 189-190
eye brows, coloring: 144
eyelash, coloring: 144

F
Faulkner, Teri: 4
finger nails: see nails

finger sculpt: 43
finger waves: 45
flakes: 53
flat iron: 74-75, 87
flexible resins: 50
foam cushion rollers: 56
Foltz, Mark: 5
Ford and Company: 5
Ford, Bill: 5
formaldehyde: 158
formaldehyde: 158
Freeman, Charlie: 5
freezing-type resins: 50
French braid: 47-48
French roll: 68
French twists: 69, 132
frizzies: 29
frosting: 140

G

gel, application: 42
gel, build-up: 11
gel, mist-type: 43
gel, non-flaking: 131
gel, spray: 39, 43-44
Glad Wrap: 31
glaze: 39, 44
glazes, vegetable: 144
Goehrke, Bob: 4
gray hair, African-Americans: 124
gray hair, brassy look: 14
gray hair, turned blue: 14

H

hair body: 41
hair breakage: 33
hair brushes: see brushes
hair build-up: 52
hair care products, professional: 9
hair care, after shampoo: 28
hair color, before the wedding: 146

hair color, blonde without bleach:
   148
hair color, chemical buffer: 147
hair color, crayons: 155
hair color, dark roots: 147, 149
hair color, differences from chart:
   156
hair color, enhancing: 14
hair color, experimenting: 145
hair color, fading: 147
hair color, fading: 154
hair color, for dirt-blond hair: 149
hair color, for dry hair: 151
hair color, for gray hair: 153, 155
hair color, for permed hair: 143
hair color, getting the green out:
   154
hair color, guidelines: 139
hair color, highlighted: 148-150
hair color, how often: 144
hair color, itchy scalp: 152
hair color, least harmful: 143
hair color, lengthening time: 155
hair color, lightened: 146-147
hair color, lightening in winter: 154
hair color, mixing colors: 152
hair color, natural look: 141
hair color, options for dark hair:
   149
hair color, options: 138
hair color, orange halo avoidance:
   147
hair color, post treatment for
   softening: 141
hair color, removal: 143
hair color, semi-permanent: 151
hair color, shelf life: 143
hair color, single process: 150
hair color, spot retouching: 155
hair color, temporary: 145-146
hair color, two-toned effect: 150
hair color, when pregnant: 152
hair conditioners: see conditioners

hair curling, non-heat rollers: see rollers
hair dryers: 22, 68, 74, 76, 78
hair dryers, bonnet-type: 77
hair dryers, convertible bonnet: 82
hair dryers, for traveling: 76-77
hair dryers, high wattage, quick drying: 79
hair dryers, with low or cool setting: 79
hair drying black hair: 136
hair ends: 40
hair extensions: 53, 132
hair highlighting, brunettes: 142
hair jewelry: 70
hair luster: 36
hair mask: 36
hair part: 43
hair pins: 69
hair removal: 192-197
hair removal: see also depilatory
hair removal, facial: 197
hair removal, nose and ears: 197
hair removal, with hand-held machine: 193
hair rinse: 35
hair static: 28
hair tangles: 29
hair texturizer: 35
hair thickener: 35
hair twirlers: 56
hair, affected by medications: 36
hair, after shampoo: 19
hair, avoiding breakage: 42
hair, blue: 14
hair, breaking off: 127
hair, brittle: 30
hair, chemically processed: 51
hair, chemically straightened: 115
hair, crown: 43
hair, damaged: 33
hair, dry, restoring: 125
hair, dry: 16

hair, dull: 46, 131
hair, dulled by tap water: 36
hair, fine: 26
hair, flat: 67
hair, flyaway: 45, 58
hair, fried from perming: 15
hair, frizzy and fly-away: 29
hair, ingrown: 194
hair, oily: 16, 18, 27
hair, over conditioned: 25
hair, over processed: 33
hair, smooth for African-Americans: 128
hair, stiff: 42
hair, stressed: 33
hair, teasing: 63
hair, thick and dull: 40
hair, thin and fine: 39
hair, what is it: 10
hair, yellow and brassy: 14
hairdressings, for African-Americans: 128
hairspray, brush out: 51
hairspray, causing hair to fall out: 51
hairspray, non-flaking: 131
hairspray, pump or aerosol: 52
hairspray, super hold: 50
hairspray, working: 50
hairspray: 49-52
Hammond, Clyde, Sr.: 5
hands, rough and red: 190
hands, softener: 190
hangnail removal: 162
Harry, Jamie: 4
Hart, Rosanne: 5
Hathaway, Carmen: 5
head wrap: 22, 31, 70
Head, Joyce: 4
headbands: 70
heat cap: 22
heat lamp: 79
Helene Curtis, Inc.: 4

henna: 121, 142
holding spray, with low alcohol: 129

Horshowski, Myra: 4
hot combs: see combs
hot oil treatment: 34
hot rollers: see rollers, hot
humectant: 24
hydrogen bonds: 94

I
Infusion 23: 26, 28
isopropyl alcohol: 24

J
jewelry, for hair: 70
Jones, Debbie: 5

K
keratin: 10

L
L'Image Salons: 4
leg waxing, at home: 194
leg waxing, ingrown hair removal: 194
leg waxing, length of hair: 193
leg waxing, pain lessening: 193
leg waxing, techniques: 194
lemon juice: 151
lemon rinse: 35
loofah: 191
lotion, thermal styling: 45
lotion, wrapping, African-Americans: 127
lotions, setting: 46

M
magnetic rollers: see rollers
manicure tools, antiseptic: 184
manicure, American: 174
manicure, breather: 160

manicure, French: 174
manicure, heat treatments: 189
manicure, in a salon: 161
manicure, preventing infection: 182
manicure, products for home use: 160
manicure, professional: 159
manicure, salon perfect at home: 161
manicure, time it should last: 160
manicure, touch up versus removal: 161
manicure, touchups: 159
Marcel iron: 83
Mast, Dayton: 4
medications affecting hair: 36
Miller, Tomarie: 5
mineral oils: 159

moisturizer, oil-based: 126
moisturizing lotion, African-Americans: 127
molded waves: 45
mousse: 11, 39-41, 52
mousse build-up: 11
mousse, after conditioning: 41
multi-toned look: 149

N
nail board, four-sided: 165
nail buffer: 166
nail color, long fingers: 173
nail color, red of short nails: 173
nail color, small hands: 173
nail disk, circular: 165
nail extensions: 179-183
nail extensions, acrylic pros and cons: 178
nail extensions, filing with glue: 183
nail extensions, sculptured acrylic: 179
nail files, emery board: 165
nail files, metal: 165

nail files, soft: 166
nail files, which to use: 164
nail fungus: 184
nail length, for the bride-to-be: 167
nail length, large, athletic hands: 167
nail length, short fingers: 166
nail polish remover, acetone: 184
nail polish remover, as conditioner: 185
nail polish remover, non-acetone: 184
nail polish, basecoat: 169
nail polish, bubbling up: 175
nail polish, drying time before typing: 176
nail polish, drying time: 175
nail polish, for special occasions: 177
nail polish, frosted: 174
nail polish, matte: 174
nail polish, nail art for a wedding: 178
nail polish, nail art: 177-178
nail polish, number of coats: 175
nail polish, opaque look: 174
nail polish, peeling off: 169
nail polish, removing smudges: 177
nail polish, sheet marks: 176
nail polish, time before bathing: 176
nail polish, topcoat: 169
nail polish, yellowing from smoking: 188
nail polish, yellowing in sunlight: 187
nail polish, yellowing in sunlight: 188
nail ridges, causes and cures: 167-168
nail strengthener: 170
nail tips and wraps: 180-181
nail wrapping: 182

nail wraps, fiberglass: 181
nail wraps, linen: 181
nail wraps, liquid: 181
nail wraps, silk: 181
nails, chipped near tips: 172
nails, gel extensions: 183
nails, greenish looking: 183
nails, growing too fast: 171
nails, growth products: 171
nails, moisturizer: 190
nails, natural: 159
nails, polish chipping: 172
nails, repairing broken ones: 189
nails, splitting: 182
nails, staying pink after polish removal: 187
nails, sunburned: 186
nails, thick and difficult to shape: 164
nails, thin as eggshells: 180
nails, week and brittle: 170

O
OrigiNails: 5
over-conditioned hair: 25
over-processing: 33

P
panthenol: 13
paraffin wrap: 190
paraffin, for hair removal: 193
pedicure, for calluses: 186
pedicure, for healthy feet: 185
pedicure, for thickened skin: 186
perm rod: 107
perm rollers: 111
perm weave: 97
perm, after shampoo: 105
perm, and color: 101
perm, before the wedding: 102
perm, bisulfate: 96
perm, blow drying: 104

perm, botanical: 106
perm, causing baldness: 104
perm, change hair color: 101
perm, chemical free: 98
perm, chemical: 106
perm, conditioning program: 109
perm, consulting stylist first: 101
perm, curly, grow out: 120
perm, dull hair: 110
perm, exothermic: 96
perm, for African-Americans: 120
perm, for falling hair: 109
perm, for fine hair: 107
perm, for hair growing out: 108
perm, for height at crown: 109
perm, for sun damaged hair: 108
perm, for swimmers: 102
perm, for thin flyaway hair: 103
perm, frizzes: 110
perm, frizzy: 99
perm, growing-out stage, survival:
    100
perm, hair condition: 103
perm, hair cutting time: 103
perm, hairspray: 110
perm, home versus professional 95
perm, how it works: 94
perm, how often: 102
perm, long lasting: 102
perm, medications affecting" 105
perm, odor: 106
perm, pageboy style: 100
perm, processing time: 94
perm, products to use after: 111
perm, redone: 99
perm, rejuvenator: 110
perm, rejuvenator: 99
perm, reverse: 97
perm, root: 96
perm, short lasting: 100
perm, spiral: 97
perm, sun parched: 105
perm, too curly: 98

perm, using a blow dryer: 104
perm, using mousse or gel with: 104
perm, wash, dry and go: 108
perm, washing hair after: 104
perm, while pregnant: 100
perm. cold wave: 106
permanent: see perm
pH: 8-9
picks: 52
picks, for relaxed hair: 133
picks, used for: 64
pin curl clips: 69
pin curls: 69
plastic mesh rollers: see rollers
polish: see nail polish
pomades: 128
ponytail: 30
pony tail holders: 70
preconditioning: 151
professional hair care products: 9
protein packs: 23
protein treatment: 29-30
psoriasis: 17
pumice stone: 189

R
ratt: 68, 132
reconstructor: 34
relaxed hair, age for use: 117
relaxed hair, chemically treated:
    120
relaxed hair, coloring: 121
relaxers: 115-120
relaxers, difference: 116
relaxers, hair regime: 118
relaxers, lye and non-lye: 116, 119
relaxers, odor: 113
relaxers, texturizing: 119
relaxers, use of: 118
relaxers, versus curl: 116
relaxers, with moisturizers: 119
relaxers, with shampoo: 119
ridge fillers, finger nails: 168

rinse temperature: see shampoo
rinse time: see shampoo
rinse-clean factor: see shampoo
roller clips, double prong: 67
roller frizzies: 68
roller pins, wire: 67
rollers, brush: 56
rollers, electric: 84
rollers, hair curling, non-heat: 65
rollers, hot build up: 90
rollers, hot direction of roll: 91
rollers, hot heat up time: 91
rollers, hot, after perm: 85
rollers, hot: 30, 35, 45, 74-75,
    88-91
rollers, jumbo: 65
rollers, magnetic: 56, 66-67
rollers, non-heat: 65-67
rollers, plastic mesh: 56
rollers, snap-on magnetic: 56
rollers, snap-on: 56
rollers, steam: 56
rollers, steam: 75, 88-89
rollers, type of: 56
rollers, Velcro: 56, 59, 64, 66
rollers, wire mesh: 56
roots, dark: 147
roots, drying: 78
round balls on hair brushes: 57

S
Sally Beauty Supply: 4, 6-7
scalp, dry: 18
scalp, itching: 34
scalp, itchy: 152
scalp, oily: 18, 24, 123
Schueller, Eugene: 139
scrunch curls: 43
SD-40 alcohol: 24
setting lotions: 46
shampoo, after deep-penetrating
    treatment: 32
shampoo, after treatment: 19

shampoo, body-building: 12
shampoo, brand usage: 11
shampoo, clarifying: 11-12, 25
shampoo, cleansing: 11
shampoo, color enhancing: 110
shampoo, color safe: 150
shampoo, dandruff: 17-18
shampoo, everyday: 10
shampoo, for African-Americans:
    124
shampoo, for build-up: 12
shampoo, for chemically treated
    hair: 17
shampoo, for color fading: 16
shampoo, for color-treated hair: 15
shampoo, for dry hair: 16
shampoo, for dry scalp: 17
shampoo, for fast hair growth: 10
shampoo, for fine, thin hair: 13
shampoo, for fried hair: 15
shampoo, for hair color enhancing:
    14
shampoo, for heavy hair lotions:
    124
shampoo, for mineral build-up: 12
shampoo, for oily, greasy hair: 16
shampoo, for permed hair: 15
shampoo, for swimmers: 18-19
shampoo, gray hair: 14
shampoo, highlighting: 14
shampoo, how often: 123
shampoo, hypo-allergenic: 15
shampoo, ingredients: 12
shampoo, lighter formula: 10
shampoo, no rinse: 17
shampoo, no-rinse: 17
shampoo, normalizing: 15, 28
shampoo, perm rejuvenating: 15
shampoo, rinse temperature: 19
shampoo, rinse time: 19
shampoo, rinse-clean factor: 12
shampoo, same brand as
    conditioner: 25

shampoo, selecting: 122
shampoo, to get rid of medications: 12
shampoo, using several brands: 11
shampoo, with botanical extracts: 13
shampoo, with natural sources: 12
shampoo, with sunscreen: 16
shaving, before going to the beach: 196
shaving, best times: 196
shaving, redness and stinging: 196
shaving, techniques: 196
shaving, the bikini area: 197
shears, for trimming: 70
sheen spray, African-Americans: 127
sheet marks, 176
shine without stiffness, African-Americans: 129
shiners: 35, 45-48
snap-on magnetic rollers: see rollers
snap-on rollers: see rollers
sodium laureth sulfate: 12
spiked styles: 46
split ends: 25, 35, 71
sponges, natural: 190
sponges, synthetic: 190
spray gel: see gel, spray
spring iron: 83
spritz: 39, 49
static, in hair: 28
steam rollers: see rollers
stearyl alcohol: 24
straightening appliances, African-Americans: 135
streaking: 140
style, reviving: 42
styling aids, African-Americans: 131
styling aids, for use with hot rollers: 45
styling products, with sunscreen: 53
styling, fine thin hair: 39
Summit Co.: 5

sun bleaching, black hair: 125
sunscreen: 19, 53, 105
surfactant: 12

T
tensile strength: 30
thermal styling lotion: 35
tipping: 140
toe nails, clipping tools: 186
toe nails, how to trim: 186
toe nails, sunburned: 186
toe nails, yellowed: 187
toluene: 174
Tong brushes: 59
trimming shears: 70
tweezers: 189-190
tweezers, causing irritation: 190
tweezers, choosing the right ones: 189
twisters, cloth: 70

U
University of North Texas: 5
upsweeps: 132

V
Velcro rollers: see rollers
Viera, James W.: 4
Vita E: 49-50
vitamin B-5: 13

W
Walker, Susan: 4
wave clamps: 43
waves, finger: 45
waves, molded: 45
wavy look, without perm: 43
waxing: see leg waxing
wet comb: 28
wet look: 44
wide-tooth comb: 52
wire mesh rollers: see rollers
wrapping lotion, African-Americans: 127

A Final Note

For product information and availability, call **1-800-284-7255**.

We invite you to send us your beauty questions for inclusion in the Second Edition of "500 Beauty Solutions." Address questions to :

Attn: 500 Beauty Solutions
The Hart Agency, Inc.
2811 McKinney Avenue, Suite 203
Dallas, TX 75204

You may enjoy these two other titles from Sourcebooks:

FINDING PEACE: Letting Go and Liking It

Finding peace in your heart is coming to terms with all that you've been through, all that you are and all that you will be. Filled with carefully crafted thoughts, suggestions, and uplifting quotes, Finding Peace gives you the opportunity to reassess how you live your life, to contemplate, to forgive, and to accept.

ISBN 1-57071-014-7; $7.95

FINDING TIME: Breathing Space for Women Who Do Too Much

Finding Time has won critical acclaim for its comprehensive, insightful, easy-to-understand tips because today's woman tends to take on too much. Finding Time will help you differentiate what should be done, what you want to do, and what you don't have to do.

ISBN 0-942061-33-0; $7.95

For these, or more copies of 500 Beauty Solutions, please contact your local bookseller, or call Sourcebooks at 1-800-SBS-8866. You may obtain a copy of our catalog by writing or faxing:

SOURCEBOOKS
P. O. Box 372, Naperville, IL 60566
(708) 961-3900
FAX: (708) 961-2168

January

1
2
3
4
5
6
7
8
9
10
11
12
13
14
15

16
17
18
19
20
21
22
23
24
25
26
27
28
29
30
31

New Hair Resolutions

• The new year is a good time to think about a transformation: a new haircut, color or perm. Magazine photos can be inspiring, but remember to consider the shape of your face, the texture and thickness of your hair and talk to your stylist.

• Ask your stylist to diagnose the condition of your hair and trim any dry, split ends. If your hair is damaged, have a deep conditioning protein treatment.

• Fight the dry frizzies of winter with a leave-in moisturizer or conditioner.

• For permed or color-treated hair, select a shampoo designed for you.

February

1
2
3
4
5
6
7
8
9
10
11
12
13
14
15

16
17
18
19
20
21
22
23
24
25
26
27
28

Valentine At-Home Spa

• Treat yourself and your loved one with a his-and-her at-home spa. It's a needed rejuvenator for your skin and an special way to show how much you care.

• Put together an enticing array of sponges, loofahs, scrubs, masks, bath gels and moisturizers for an afternoon of clean fun!

• For a romantic evening at home, try soaking in a candlelight herb- or flower-scented bath. Don't forget some soft, relaxing music to help set the mood. Then give each other a back or foot massage using a soothing oil or refreshing foot gel.

March

1		16
2		17
3		18
4		19
5		20
6		21
7		22
8		23
9		24
10		25
11		26
12		27
13		28
14		29
15		30
		31

Handle with Care

• As winter winds down, get a jump on spring with a professional manicure, a paraffin treatment to soften hands and cuticles and a snappy, new nail polish color!

• If nail ridges are a problem, use a ridge filler as a base coat or experiment with buffing your nails for smooth, shining, natural nails.

• Because moisture loss is a major cause of nail brittleness and breakage, moisturize hands daily and use a cuticle conditioner to help stimulate healthy growth and fight the drying effects of wintery cold and indoor heat.

April

1		16
2		17
3		18
4		19
5		20
6		21
7		22
8		23
9		24
10		25
11		26
12		27
13		28
14		29
15		30

Spring Cleaning

• Toss out old makeup and applicators to prevent bacteria build-up! Restock cotton swabs, cosmetic wedges, sponges, eye makeup applicators, and powder puffs.

• Wash your combs and brushes and clean electronic hair tools according to manufacturers instructions. Replace old makeup brushes; throw away hair brushes that have lost their protective tips.

• Check your nail supplies: Discard old polish and files. When purchasing files, remember the higher the grit number, the smoother the file. Sanitize your manicure tools.

May

1		16
2		17
3		18
4		19
5		20
6		21
7		22
8		23
9		24
10		25
11		26
12		27
13		28
14		29
15		30
		31

May Makeover

• Summer's coming, so uncover your best assets.

• To enliven your skin, give your self a home facial, using a mask for your skin type, followed by a toner and moisturizer. Or pamper yourself with a professional salon facial.

• Sun exposure can damage and prematurely age your skin. Be sure to use skin products with SP 15 or higher.

• If smooth summer legs are your priority, begin regular leg and bikini waxing. If shaving is your hair removal method, try using hair conditioner as a shaving cream for silky, soft results.

June

1		16
2		17
3		18
4		19
5		20
6		21
7		22
8		23
9		24
10		25
11		26
12		27
13		28
14		29
15		30

Footloose

• Baring your feet won't embarrass you if you begin with a professional pedicure. The foot massage will revitalize your weary feet and a fresh coat of bright polish will perk up your spirits.

• Every time you bathe, remove dry skin and calluses with a pumice stone, a foot file or a special sloughing lotion. Finish with a cooling powder or icy foot gel.

• Moisturize your feet daily.

• Prevent natural nails or light-colored polish from yellowing with a topcoat containing an ultra violet inhibitor.

July

1		16
2		17
3		18
4		19
5		20
6		21
7		22
8		23
9		24
10		25
11		26
12		27
13		28
14		29
15		30
		31

Summer Tress Distress

• Salt water and chlorine can weigh down and dry out your hair. Remove ocean or pool water with special swimmers' shampoos that both clarify and moisturize your hair.

• To keep hair from drying out or fading in the summer sun, use styling products with sunscreens to help protect hair from the sun's damaging UV rays.

• Use a wide-tooth comb on clean, wet hair. A leave-in conditioner will prevent breakage and add sheen.

• For split ends, trim and condition hair regularly and try a silicone based hair shiner for instant results.

August

1		16
2		17
3		18
4		19
5		20
6		21
7		22
8		23
9		24
10		25
11		26
12		27
13		28
14		29
15		30
		31

Color Care

• When coloring your hair for the first time, ask your salon stylist to make a subtle change and help you choose a color close to your natural shade. Or, try a temporary color to ensure the right shade.

• For dry hair that needs color, precondition with a deep-penetrating moisturizing or protein treatment.

• Extend the life of your new hair color with a clear color gloss, which seals the cuticle and leaves hair healthy and shiny.

• To brighten fading hair color, use a color-enhancing shampoo designed to freshen or tone the hair.

September

1		16
2		17
3		18
4		19
5		20
6		21
7		22
8		23
9		24
10		25
11		26
12		27
13		28
14		29
15		30

A Season for Change

• Fall marks the fashion new year, a time when we yearn for change.
• To achieve smoother styles with curly hair, use a styling comb designed to straighten or style coarse, thick hair.
• If your hair is fine and thin, a body wave will provide needed curve and volume.
• For a tight wavy look without a perm, use a hot crimping iron.
• Relaxing or straightening hair requires powerful chemicals. Consult your stylist for best results.
• For a fast, dry set, spray hair with gel, use Velcro® rollers and blow dry.

October

1		16
2		17
3		18
4		19
5		20
6		21
7		22
8		23
9		24
10		25
11		26
12		27
13		28
14		29
15		30
		31

A Flawless Facade

• Blending is the key to beautiful make-up. Be sure you have the right tools!
• Blend foundation outward with a damp cosmetic sponge or wedge.
• Outline your lips with a lip pencil or lip brush. Soften the line with a cotton swab and apply color with the flat side of the lip brush.
• Apply subtle eye color with a flat eyeshadow brush.
• For a natural looking glow, apply blush with a large, soft blush brush, blending upward and outward.
• Set your makeup with translucent powder, applied with a large powder brush or velour powder puff.

November

1	16
2	17
3	18
4	19
5	20
6	21
7	22
8	23
9	24
10	25
11	26
12	27
13	28
14	29
15	30

Flake Off!

- Dry scalp, caused by drying heat and/or overuse of chemicals, can cause flakes, too. A moisturizing or dry scalp shampoo will help.
- If you are a daily user of styling products, such as mousse or gel, use a clarifying shampoo once a week to eliminate flakes caused by product build-up.
- Fight oily dandruff flakes with dandruff shampoos containing special ingredients that shake dandruff loose.
- Remember, if you suspect a medical skin condition, such as eczema or psoriasis, consult your doctor or dermatologist.

December

1	16
2	17
3	18
4	19
5	20
6	21
7	22
8	23
9	24
10	25
11	26
12	27
13	28
14	29
15	30
	31

Holiday Hints

- To enhance your natural hair color, try a highlighting shampoo with a vegetable dye to add depth and subtle shading.
- For festive nail effects, nail art is the answer! Now anyone can create lacey or colorful foil designs with decal kits. But be sure to follow all directions carefully.
- To hold that special holiday hair style for hours, use a styling glaze before you style or a freezing hair spray after you style your hair.
- Between day and evening, reactivate the gel in your hair with a spritz of leave-in conditioner, then restyle.